PRAISE FOR *ANTIDEP*

"...a valuable input to the process of change in global mental health and an essential book for both users and providers of mental health services."

—Dainius Pūras, MD,
Professor of Child and Adolescent Psychiatry and former UN Special Rapporteur on the Right to Health

"...vital to understanding SSRIs and other antidepressants."

—Will Hall, MA,
author of *The Harm Reduction Guide to Coming Off Psychiatric Drugs*

"...essential reading for anyone prescribing or taking antidepressants."

—Marion Brown, BSc, MBA, HG.Dip.P

"...a book every medical professional should read."

—Jill Nickens,
founder of Akathisia Alliance

"...provides a summary of what you need to know which has been difficult to access before now."

—Dr. Sian F. Gordon, MBChB, MRCGP

"...a powerful examination of the potential consequences of an overtly medical response to emotional distress."

—James Moore,
host of the Let's Talk Withdrawal and Mad in America podcasts

ANTIDEPRESSED

ANTIDEPRESSED

A BREAKTHROUGH EXAMINATION OF EPIDEMIC ANTIDEPRESSANT HARM AND DEPENDENCE

BEVERLEY THOMSON

Hatherleigh Press is committed to preserving and protecting the natural resources of the earth. Environmentally responsible and sustainable practices are embraced within the company's mission statement.

Visit us at www.hatherleighpress.com and register online for free offers, discounts, special events, and more.

ANTIDEPRESSED

Text Copyright © 2021 Beverley Thomson

Library of Congress Cataloging-in-Publication Data is available.
ISBN: 978-1-57826-923-5

All rights reserved. No part of this book may be reproduced, stored in a retrieval system, or transmitted, in any form or by any means, electronic or otherwise, without written permission from the publisher.

Printed in the United States
10 9 8 7 6 5 4 3 2 1

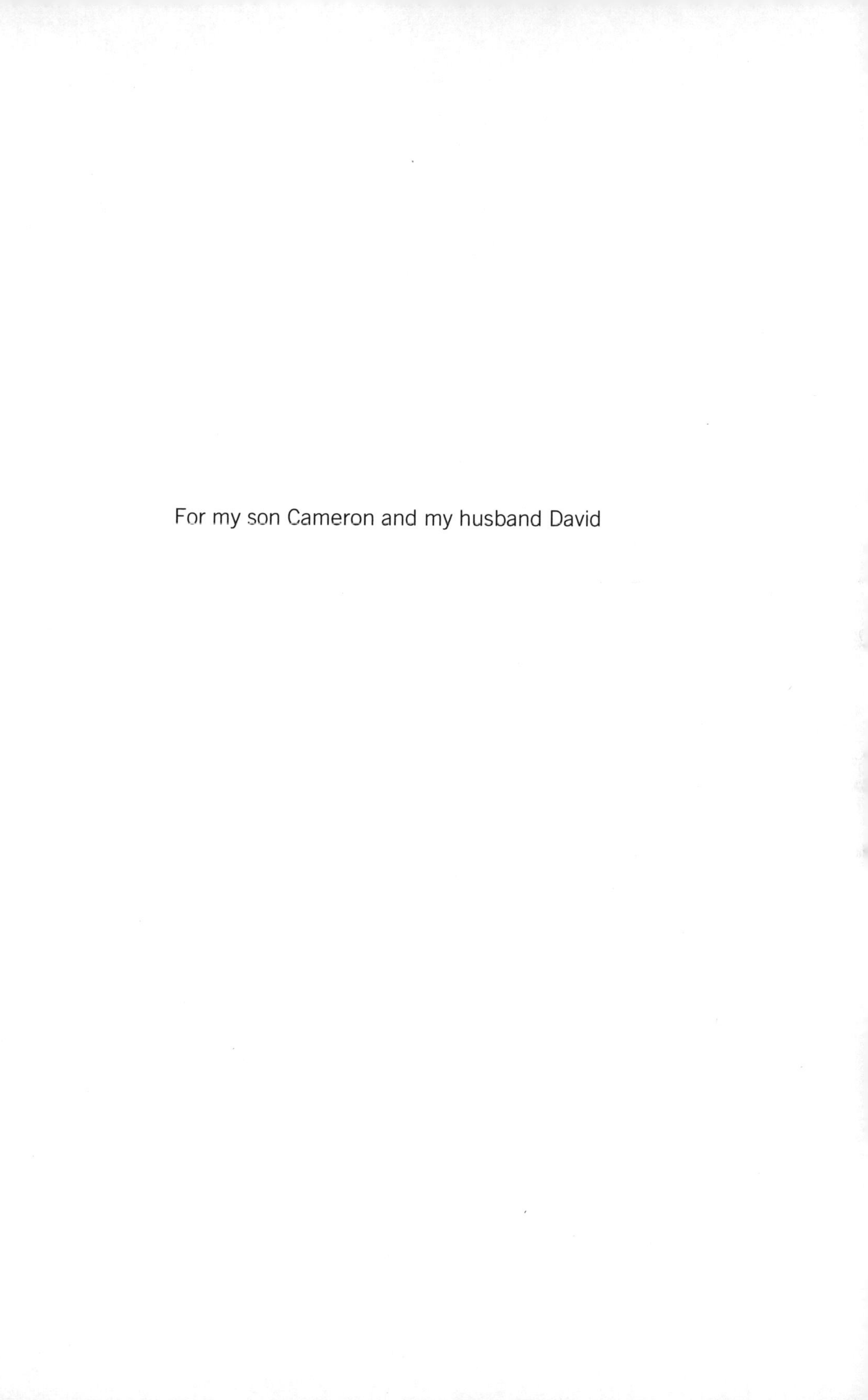

For my son Cameron and my husband David

CONTENTS

Preface xi

Introduction: Our "Wicked" Problem with Antidepressants xiii

PART 1

The Medicalization of Our Mental Health and Antidepressant Prescribing 1

1: How Our Mental Health Became Medical 3

2: The Myth of the Chemical Imbalance 8

3: The Unrecognized Power of the Pill 11

4: Mental Health:The Business 14

PART 2

The Power of the Informed Patient 19

5: Alternatives Worth Considering 21

6: Being Informed About Our Treatment Options 24

7: The Importance of Informed Consent 26

8: Knowing Antidepressant Benefits and Risks 32

9: The Many Adverse Effects Including Akathisia 41

10: Antidepressant-Induced Suicide 63

11: Antidepressants and Our "Medically Unexplained Symptoms" 71

12: Becoming Our Own Antidepressant Expert 78

13: Antidepressant Long-Term Effects 80

14: Dependence and Our New Balanced State 88
15: Withdrawal: The Relapse Trap and Research 93

PART 3

Safe Antidepressant Management and Withdrawal 107
16: Adopting a Harm Reduction Approach 109
17: Learning About Our Antidepressants and Listening to Our Body 112
18: Withdrawal and the Existing Professional Advice 119

PART 4

Special Concerns 125
19: Same But Not The Same: Understanding Generics 127
20: Prescribing Antidepressants to Children and Young People 131
21: The Elderly, Vulnerability and Antidepressants 138
22: Antidepressants, the Armed Forces, PTSD and Suicide 142

PART 5

Patient Experiences 149

CONCLUSION 239

THE RESOURCE GUIDE 246
Useful Resources 248
Additional Reading 265
Key Articles, Information and Research 270
Acknowledgments 284
References 286

PREFACE

Dear Dr. Gordon,

I have been suffering from extremely severe withdrawal symptoms from the antidepressant drug paroxetine for over six months now. These symptoms include but are not limited to: body and head jerking, severe agitation, hyperventilation to the point of passing out, and waves of "toxic depression".

I admitted myself to hospital after a failed attempt to take my own life. They discharged me after 10 days as there was nothing they could do for/with me and I was becoming a burden on the nurses and the other patients.

Every second of my waking existence is horrific. I have repeatedly expressed my wish to die with dignity as I am now unable to maintain even the most basic standards of personal hygiene. I have socially isolated to the extreme as my condition makes associating with people impossible.

In my desperate state I have contacted the group "My Death My Decision" as well as the group "Exit International" so they will have a record of my experience even though there is nothing they can do to help me.

You have my permission to share my correspondence with anyone you deem to be appropriate.

Yours sincerely,

Antony Schofield

THIS BOOK COMES too late for Antony Schofield. He ended his life aged 52. Being prescribed antidepressants was the start of a ruined and wasted life. I talk with his mother often; at 81, she was left with only memories of a wonderful, intelligent and adventurous son. Antony's mum is now aware of and understands the effects these drugs, taken as prescribed, had on her son's life. It was Antony's wish, and is now his mother's, that people should learn about the harm these medications have the potential to cause. Towards the end of his suffering, he asked his mother to "tell the world" about antidepressants. This book is the voice of Antony and his mum Bridget.

INTRODUCTION

Our "Wicked" Problem with Antidepressants

"Wicked'" refers to a problem that cannot be fixed, where there is no single solution to the problem. "Wicked" denotes resistance to resolution, rather than evil. Another definition is "a problem whose social complexity means that it has no determinable stopping point and because of complex interdependencies, the effort to solve one aspect of a "wicked" problem may reveal or create other problems."[1]

NOWADAYS, WE TALK about the urgent need for a paradigm shift in how we think about mental health and for "transformation in the way we collectively understand and intervene on mental health issues."[2] The reality is we need a revolution. In 2020, the United Nations published a report[3] by Special Rapporteur Dainius Pūras calling for "little short of a revolution in mental health care."[4]

It is important to remember, whatever we need to do to make change and however loud we shout about emerging new ways of thinking, antidepressant prescribing is continuing to soar around the world. The medicalized way we look at mental health has become a dominant and powerful one and millions of us have chosen to take antidepressants knowing very little about them. Whilst the medical profession has a responsibility to "first do no harm," we, as patients also have a responsibility to learn about this medication we take, often with very little thought. It is hoped that this book will enable us to become savvy about antidepressants, make informed choices and contribute to changing how we think about, talk about, and cope with life's up and downs.

Mental "illnesses" are amongst the most common health conditions in the United States.

- More than 50% will be diagnosed with a mental illness or disorder at some point in their lifetime.
- 1 in 5 Americans will experience a mental illness in a given year.
- 1 in 5 children, either currently or at some point during their life, have had a seriously debilitating mental illness.
- 1 in 25 Americans lives with a serious mental illness, such as schizophrenia, bipolar disorder, or major depression.[5]

The US has declared itself to be in the grips of a mental health epidemic. According to Centers for Disease Control and Prevention (CDC) data, one in seven—or 13.2 percent—of adults aged 18 and over took antidepressants between 2015 and 2018; more than 43 million adults. Use was higher amongst women, 17.7 percent, than men, 8.4 percent. This increased with age, rising to 24.3 percent of all women aged 60 and above. Teenagers, aged 13–19, experienced the greatest increase in antidepressant use from 2015 to 2019, up a significant 38.3 percent, from 5.7 percent to 7.9 percent.[6,7] This significant rise in use amongst young people is alarming. One study reports the number of young people with major depression jumped 52 percent between 2005 and 2017. In addition, 1 in 8 young Americans now suffers from anxiety.[8]

This is written at the time of COVID-19 and already in the US there have been significant increases in the prescribing of drugs used to treat mental health conditions. Statistics for 2020 show 45 million Americans were taking antidepressants and this included 2.1 million young people aged 0–17. By March 2020, it was reported prescriptions for antidepressants had risen by 19 percent, anti-anxiety medication by 34 percent and anti-insomnia drugs by 15 percent. Reports tell of 40 million Americans suffering from anxiety and over 17 million being diagnosed with Major Depressive Disorder.[9]

The American Psychiatric Association (APA) Practice Guideline for the Treatment of Patients with Major Depressive Disorder recommends antidepressants or psychotherapy as the initial treatment for patients with mild-to-moderate depression.[10] Yet financial costs prevent many Americans accessing medication or therapy. It is also reported there is a severe lack of mental health professionals available with a shortage of counsellors, social workers, psychiatrists and psychologists. Only one-third of those diagnosed receive treatment because of the cost of care, according to the Anxiety and Depression Association of America.[11] The U.S. Department of Health and Human Services says approximately 111 million Americans live in areas with a shortage of mental health professionals.[12]

Despite prescription statistics, there has never been any sound evidence for the epidemic of depression talked about. We do, however, have a mental health pseudo epidemic in the western world and the case of an epidemic of antidepressant prescribing is a reality. The surge in antidepressant prescribing has always been a growing cultural trend as well as a medical one. It reflects the rise of the "medicalization" of everyday life and is one which comes at a cost to individuals and society. Unfortunately, the promotion of "mental health" as medical conditions has led, primarily, to the increase in the prescribing of antidepressants and it is now becoming widely recognized that antidepressants can put us at risk of dangerous adverse effects; most notably they can cause dependence and raise the risk of suicide. It is also ironic that as antidepressant prescribing continues to soar, so does mental health disability.[13]

Dependence on antidepressants is an issue lacking much needed recognition; a worldwide "elephant in the room," and for many it can be personally, socially, or politically uncomfortable to deal with. It can be embarrassing, controversial, inflammatory, and downright dangerous. The pharmaceutical industry, psychiatry and doctors are supported by governments and mental health organizations and charities in propagating the unsubstantiated basis on which mental health has grown to be a huge industry. They have made antidepressants the medication so many of us have come to depend on. Many of us claim antidepressants have saved our lives, but many are unaware of the harm antidepressants have caused or of our dependence on the medication we take as prescribed.

Just as happened with the campaigns in the 1990s, the drug companies will no doubt seize the potential COVID-19 presents as an opportunity to capture new customers, expand existing mental health markets, and introduce their medical model of treatment to new ones. In the 1990s, Eli Lilly and the field of psychiatry created an incredibly successful epidemic of pseudo-depression. By 2000, Prozac had 40 million users and accounted for a quarter of Eli Lilly's $10.8 billion sales and more than a third of its $3 billion profit. Before Prozac arrived, the general public were against antidepressants and believed them addictive.

Media language during COVID-19 is serving to assist the pharmaceutical industry to further boost its profits during and in the aftermath of the crisis. This is a time when language matters and we must be aware of similar campaigns to "Defeat Depression" and "Depression Hurts;" crusades which in the 1990s led to the unsubstantiated medicating of our mental health and to millions today being dependent on and harmed by antidepressants.[14] It is important we are not duped into falling for a well-orchestrated "Defeat COVID-19 Mental Illness Campaign" or "COVID-19 PTSD Campaign," which are probably already in the planning stage. The future mental health of a generation now depends on the powerful language used to help us cope with our lives during this time.

Overtreatment with antidepressants and underestimation of risks have left millions around the world with problems to which there are no obvious solutions. Current levels of antidepressant prescribing are unsustainable for many reasons. It is a human time-bomb, sometimes fueled by the willful blindness of both patients and medical professionals. Failure to acknowledge the issues is leading to harm and death and when the issue of dependence is raised, other problems present themselves due to the lack of research, knowledge, and existing support for those who choose to withdraw from antidepressants.

Vulnerability is hardly ever spoken about in relation to antidepressants and yet, it is the one adverse effect we will most probably be prescribed with our medication. We can be vulnerable to physical and psychological adverse effects and vulnerable when dependence causes changes to our health, sometimes leading to many aspects of our life spiraling out of control.

This book acknowledges a problem too complex to solve but offers an opportunity to learn, open minds and explore options to avoid and reduce harm and dependence. People, right now, need help and there is little available. In an ideal world we talk about "withdrawal" from antidepressants but for many, managing their antidepressants has become a process of damage limitation. Mental illness is not a disease but is described as an epidemic and unless we challenge the current mental health narrative—unless we educate ourselves and learn about the powerful drugs we take, we will see more suffering, illness and death.[15]

Taking an antidepressant is an individual's choice. I hope this book is one people will refer to when making the choice to start taking antidepressants and whilst taking them or considering reducing or managing their medication. It is honest and straight forward about the realities of the effects of Selective Serotonin Reuptake Inhibitors (SSRIs) and Serotonin Norepinephrine Reuptake Inhibitors (SNRIs).

Taking an antidepressant should be our informed choice based on the benefits and risks. There are things it is important we know about SSRI/SNRI antidepressants and things we need to look at differently. The reality is there are many things we still don't know about these drugs. What we are told about an antidepressant will initially depend on our prescriber, but only some will be knowledgeable and honest; that it seems impossible to predict how our mind and body will react to the medication.

There is now so much information available in books and online resources about the benefits and adverse effects of antidepressants. Some information is reliable and easily accessible but for many it can appear complex and daunting. I explain the realities of the "wicked" issue of antidepressants by presenting evidence-based facts and real-life experiences. I have known too many people who wish they had been fully aware, before they swallowed their first pill, of the realities of a life "Antidepressed".

This book does not contain medical advice! It encourages and helps us learn about SSRI/SNRI antidepressants and guides us to appropriate resources enabling us to make more informed choices. The resource section of this book includes valuable sources of information including websites, books, articles, and research.

WARNING: There are many reasons why it is important that we never stop taking or start withdrawing antidepressants or any psychotropic medication without the support of a knowledgeable medical professional or support service. Antidepressant treatment should be supported by frequent reviews. We need to be aware, from the very first pill we take, of any physical or psychological changes we experience and report them immediately to our prescriber. Evidence suggests the risk of suicide, self-harm or other severe adverse events is significantly higher when commencing, stopping or changing doses or switching drugs including generics.

This book includes petition extracts from people around the world. The petition called for the Scottish Parliament to urge the Scottish Government to take action to appropriately recognise and effectively support individuals affected and harmed by prescribed drug dependence and withdrawal.[1]

In this book, "antidepressants" refers to SSRI/SNRI antidepressants unless otherwise stated.

SELECTIVE SEROTONIN REUPTAKE INHIBITORS (SSRIs)	
GENERICS	**BRAND NAMES***
Citalopram	Celexa, Cipramil
Escitalopram	Cipralex, Lexapro
Fluoxetine	Prozac, Sarafem
Fluvoxamine	Luvox, Faverin
Paroxetine	Paxil, Seroxat
Sertraline	Zoloft, Lustral

SEROTONIN NOREPINEPHRINE REUPTAKE INHIBITORS (SNRIs)	
GENERICS	**BRAND NAMES***
Desvenlafaxine	Pristiq
Duloxetine	Cymbalta
Levomilnacipran	Fetzima
Milnacipran	Ixel, Savella
Venlafaxine	Effexor
Sertraline	Zoloft, Lustral
**These drugs have many different brand names throughout the world. Medications might be available in tablet, capsule, or liquid form.*	

PART 1

The Medicalization of Our Mental Health and Antidepressant Prescribing

1
HOW OUR MENTAL HEALTH BECAME MEDICAL

Why do so many of us believe we might be "mentally ill" and need medication? Why have we been made to believe "mental health" is a medical issue?

We are told our mental health deserves parity with our physical health. Campaigns by often self-serving organizations have encouraged the developed world to see mental health as being part of our medical system. Reality is, physical health treatment is targeted at the biological cause of an illness, but mental health treatment should be primarily about helping us cope with the many personal and societal factors negatively affecting our ability to cope with our lives. Nowadays, however, it seems to suit both doctors and patients to readily accept medication as the answer rather than address the issues causing our stress, anxiety or sadness.

Something is probably wrong, difficult, uncomfortable, or downright hard in our life but millions of us are not actually "mentally ill". Psychiatry and the pharmaceutical industry have created a system of mental health to attempt to reflect diagnostic models used in other areas of medicine. This is to justify psychiatry's status as a medical profession and the prescribing of antidepressants and other psychiatric medications.

Most of us have never heard of the Diagnostic and Statistical Manual of Mental Disorders or the "DSM" as it is known. The 5th edition of this manual, (DSM–5), was published in 2013 following work groups creating hundreds of papers and articles to provide the world with a summary of the state of the supposed "science" relating to "psychiatric diagnoses". This current edition of psychiatry's bible lists over 300 disorders or illnesses for which we are likely to be prescribed antidepressants or other psychotropic medication. It is perhaps the most powerful and influential book we have probably never heard of.[16,17,18]

Using this manual as their justification, our doctors are taught to categorize our emotional feelings and subjectively and often inaccurately diagnose us as suffering from disorders and conditions. These are not biological diseases and there are no proven biological causes, but it has led to a cultural perception that depression, grief, sadness, anxiety and other normal human feelings and behaviors should be classified as mental illness. Psychiatry's classifications have become part of our culture and encouraged us to accept our suffering and inability to cope as mental health issues needing medical treatment .

The DSM categories are labels and patients are matched to them using the opinion of the doctor listening to the patient's own feelings about themselves when asked certain questions. This is not a scientific process and has many flaws; are we always being honest with the doctor and is the doctor always asking the right questions and listening correctly? Do we feel exactly the same from one day to the next? Are there reasons we think a diagnosis will make life easier? A doctor's often subconscious reference to conditions created for this "guidebook" is for many of us the start of our feelings and emotions being defined as mental illness, antidepressants or other drugs being prescribed, and the real-life issues we need to address being ignored.

Without us even recognizing it, psychiatry's DSM has become a dominant part of how we deal with everyday life. Whether we have heard of the DSM of not, its conditions have become part of our everyday language. A doctor will probably not even refer to it, but we have allowed it to mislabel normal emotions and feelings and encourage both overdiagnosis and inappropriate use of medication. There now seems to be a pill for every emotional situation we might find ourselves in and a label for every inconvenient or uncomfortable feeling. The covert DSM has been cleverly and unceremoniously drilled into our psyche and until very recently we have generally accepted it without question.

Ultimately, unless we are informed and question their opinion, whether or not we end up on medication is often decided by little more than a doctor's subjective diagnosis. Many of us who could quickly improve with time, the support of friends and family or therapy, might not be given the right sort of help we need. A doctor's appointment is often the start of a lifelong journey as a psychiatric patient resulting in a stigmatizing lifelong condition and dependence on psychiatric medication.

Is there any wonder we have come to believe "a pill" can make life easier? Why do so many of us turn to antidepressants to help us cope with life's difficulties?

Prozac (and the language that came with it) changed everything.

"Defeat Depression" and "Depression Hurts" campaigns became some of the most influential and successful marketing campaigns of our era. We suddenly had mental health and mental illness and the simple solution was to be found in a psychotropic drug branded "Prozac".[27]

Prozac, the first SSRI antidepressant was introduced in 1988. Eli Lilly marketed it as "happiness in a blister pack". Prozac, generic/medical name fluoxetine, was quickly given to Interbrand, the world's leading branding company and it was given its identity. Over the following years, national campaigns informed doctors and the public of the dangers of depression.[28]

Prozac was pushed as a wonder drug, entirely safe, an easy answer to "the blues". It fixed our faulty brains. On launch day patients were already asking for it by name. And with powerful marketing we were brainwashed into believing depression was a biological disease, chemical imbalances needed balancing and everything could easily be cured by a drug. A new kind of depressed patient was "created" and they had mild depression needing medical treatment. They were the ordinary people with ordinary life struggles and were sold the idea that a drug could make their life better.

Campaigns assessed public attitudes towards depression to discover which of them "needed" to be changed. Eli Lilly then began changing the public's opinion about antidepressants. Conclusions were made "Doctors have an important role in educating the public about depression and the rationale for antidepressant treatment." In 1997, Eli Lilly ran a new marketing campaign for Prozac with direct-to-consumer advertising. Advertisements appeared in over 20 general-interest magazines and targeted both adults who suffered from depression and their family and friends. Their target market was the new, first-time depressed patient and their messages were "Depression Hurts" and "Prozac can Help".

Initially, The American Medical Association (AMA) were not overly enthusiastic about Eli Lilly's strategy, "Of course, doctors can—and should—say no to anyone who doesn't need a particular medication. But let's not fool ourselves: If doctors are under pressure from their patients to prescribe a particular medication, they must become strong gatekeepers to prevent misuse."[29] At this time there was no internet and we relied on doctors and the pharmaceutical company's Patient Information Leaflet for information and advice. There were no social media groups for support if we needed it. We became guinea pigs in the new medicalized way of dealing with life. It was nothing short of the start of a worldwide unauthorized human experiment which continues today, unabated.

In the TIME Magazine 2003 article "If everyone was on Prozac…", Dr. Sanjay Gupta asked, "[T]hat raises an intriguing question about the future of mood-altering pharmaceuticals: If Prozac can make you feel better even if you are not depressed, why shouldn't we all be taking it? Is that the direction we're going, as the drugs become more socially acceptable and heavily marketed? (More than 11 million Americans already take some form of antidepressant.) It's a question that arises only because SSRIs are relatively mild and subtle medications. There are plenty of drugs that can make you feel better, at least temporarily—alcohol and heroin come immediately to mind—but they tend to be addictive or toxic or both. Prozac is neither."[30]

We now know antidepressants can be highly toxic and probably cause dependence for the majority of those who take them. The pharmaceutical industry and psychiatry are supported by governments, the medical profession, the media and mental health organizations and charities to continue to promote the unsubstantiated basis on which mental health has grown to be a huge industry and these drugs are "sold" to us. The clever marketing of Prozac assisted the birth of the "medical model" of mental health and we adopted it, until recently, without question.

2
THE MYTH OF THE CHEMICAL IMBALANCE

We are told it's our "chemical imbalance", but where's the proof? Why don't we have tests or scans to confirm this imbalance?

There are no biological tests such as blood tests or brain scans which can be used to provide independent objective data to support our mental health diagnosis. We have all probably heard of and believed in the "chemical imbalance" theory or that we might have "it" because we are predisposed genetically; "my mother suffered from it" or "it runs in the family".

Despite everything we might have been told about chemical imbalances, there are no known biological causes for any of the psychiatric and mental health disorders or illnesses apart from dementia and some rare chromosomal disorders.[31] We are being medically treated for conditions which are most probably not biological.

By means of the carefully scripted pharmaceutical marketing campaigns of the 1990s and pushed by psychiatry, our doctors quickly learned to attribute mental illness to faulty brain biochemistry, defects of dopamine, or a shortage of serotonin. They bought into it, we bought into it and most of us still believe it now. For over 30 years we have all been conditioned to believe what is now starting to be regarded as very questionable science. Research has mostly shown evidence that the brain, which has around 100 billion neurons and is one of the most complex objects in the universe is in fact an elusive target for drugs. It is just way too complicated for it to be as simple as we are led to believe.

From an early age we are taught "doctor knows best". Most of us trust, without question, that our doctors adhere to their principle of "first do no harm". We have accepted without question their story that our brain chemistry is at fault and these false perceptions of how our brains work have made it easy for us to accept that we might be mentally ill, and antidepressants are the answer. The fact is there are no associations with any biological pathology in relation to the majority of psychiatric diagnoses. Conditions which have become part of our everyday language such as bipolar disorder, depressive disorders, anxiety disorders, personality disorders, obsessive compulsive disorders or post-traumatic stress disorders have no associations with any biological pathology.

There is an absence of scientific evidence to support the supposed "chemical imbalance" theory and many eminent professionals are now openly questioning the validity of the theory. It is now being described as last-century thinking, misleading and unscientific "biobabble".

Although scientists have been testing the chemical imbalance theory's validity for over forty years and despite thousands of studies, there is still not one piece of direct evidence proving the theory correct. The chemical imbalance theory, in relation to any mental health disorder is unsubstantiated.

This chemical imbalance story, countlessly repeated on antidepressant commercials and by psychiatrists from prestigious institutions, has been so effective that it comes as a surprise to many Americans—including Alix Spiegel—to discover that the psychiatric establishment now claims that it has always known that this theory was not true or "urban legend," the term used by Ronald Pies, Editor-in-Chief Emeritus of the Psychiatric Times. Pies stated in 2011, "In truth, the 'chemical imbalance' notion was always a kind of urban legend—never a theory seriously propounded by well-informed psychiatrists."

Truly well-informed psychiatrists have long known that research showed that low serotonin (or other neurotransmitter) levels were not the cause of depression. The 1998 American Medical Association Essential Guide to Depression stated: "The link between low levels of serotonin and depressive illness is unclear, as some depressed people have too much serotonin. But the vast majority of Americans—who didn't read this textbook—never heard this."[32]

The American Psychiatric Association website gives the following information regarding the association between depression and brain chemistry which they say "may" exist; "Medication: Brain chemistry may contribute to an individual's depression and may factor into their treatment. For this reason, antidepressants might be prescribed to help modify one's brain chemistry."[33]

So why do we still buy into mental health being a medical issue? For many of us a doctor's or psychiatrist's diagnosis validates the way we both feel and act. It can be easier to blame our faulty brain chemistry rather than dealing with our difficult life; "It's not me it's my Bipolar, Depression, OCD, GAD", or whatever condition we have been given to justify taking medication. It sometimes makes it easier to explain why we are not coping. For some, it enables a sense of belonging, almost a cultural acceptance. But continuing to believe the chemical imbalance theory and taking drugs we don't need or understand can have life changing, often irreversible effects on us physically and psychologically. Just as importantly, blaming our brain chemistry and convincing us we need medication allows those who should be improving our social conditions and quality of life, (often the real causes of our distress), to avoid responsibility. The chemical imbalance theory has been a political and commercial no-brainer.

3
THE UNRECOGNIZED POWER OF THE PILL

Why don't we question the potential effects of taking antidepressants? Why do so many of us take these drugs knowing so little about the effects they might have on our mind and body?

Antidepressants are psychiatric drugs. They are psychoactive psychotropic substances. Psychoactive means they affect the mind, but they do so much more than simply affecting our mind. "A psychoactive drug or psychotropic substance is a chemical substance that acts primarily upon the central nervous system where it alters brain function, resulting in temporary changes in perception, mood, consciousness and behavior."[34] Most of us take antidepressants without acknowledging or being aware they are powerful psychotropic drugs and very often without going near psychiatry.

Dr. Candace Pert, the neuroscientist and pharmacologist whose work was key to the development of SSRI antidepressants spoke out against them in October 1997 in TIME magazine. "I am alarmed at the monster that Johns Hopkins neuroscientist Solomon Snyder and I created when we discovered the simple binding assay for drug receptors 25 years ago. The public is being misinformed about the precision of these selective serotonin-uptake inhibitors when the medical profession oversimplifies their action in the brain."[35]

In a 1996 paper, the National Institute of Mental Health (NIMH) director Stephen Hyman described how psychiatric medication works, "The drugs are better understood as agents that create abnormalities in brain function. Psychotropic drugs, all perturb normal neurotransmitter activity in the brain. The brain, however, has various feedback mechanisms to monitor its neurotransmitter activity, and in response to the drug's perturbation of its normal functioning, it goes through a series of "compensatory adaptations." The brain is seeking to maintain its normal functioning. The immediate molecular targets of these drugs in the nervous system initiate perturbations that activate homeostatic mechanisms... until cellular signaling reaches an adapted state which may be qualitatively and quantitatively different from the normal state."[36]

The shocking fact is, antidepressants do not cure our non-existing chemical imbalance, they actually create one and this imbalance can affect us mentally and physically. Just like other substances that affect brain chemistry (such as illicit drugs), psychiatric drugs produce altered mental states. They do not "cure" diseases, and in many cases their mechanism of action is not properly understood.[37] What we do know is they can induce varied and unpredictable mental and physical states. These drugs work more like substances that temporarily alter our state of mind, such as caffeine or cannabis. In other words, they don't cure us they simply change us. Anecdotal evidence tells us they can throw us temporarily into a foreign state of mind, into an altered version of who we are which can result in behavior and personality changes.

In terms of changing us physically, what most of us don't realize is antidepressants act directly on the central nervous system (CNS). They interfere with the functioning of the most basic and essential autonomic (sympathetic and parasympathetic) nervous systems which control all our vital functions of the body (digestive, cardiovascular, respiratory, endocrine, sleep, reproductive, immune and other systems) as well as affecting moods, feelings and complex human thought processes. We have known for many years antidepressant neurotoxicity causes neurological problems and these include movement disorders, seizures, balance and visual issues which are often diagnosed as Medically Unexplained Symptoms (MUS), Myalgic Encephalomyelitis (ME), Chronic Fatigue Syndrome (CFS) or Functional Neurological Disorder (FND).[38,39,40]

Antidepressants might create serious altered mental states and physical states so is it worth the risk? Studies have found that "antidepressants have no clinically significant benefit over placebo pills in the treatment of mild to moderate depression."[41] For around 85 percent of us, antidepressants work, on average, no better than placebo pills. This conclusion has been demonstrated by numerous meta-analyses studies which gathered together all of the clinical trials which have attempted to assess whether antidepressants work better than placebo pills. They concluded antidepressants are no more effective than placebos for most people.[42] A further, major meta-analysis commissioned by the UK NHS, and published in The Lancet, showed the difference between placebos and antidepressants is so modest, that for mild to moderate depression antidepressants were not worth having at all. As the lead author of the study stated: "Our widespread comparative meta-analysis of antidepressants showed, pretty clearly, that the difference between the published and unpublished studies of antidepressants in children, was that for the published trials, all the drugs worked, while for the unpublished trials none of the drugs worked."[43]

Professor Irving Kirsch, Harvard Medical School, conducted the most noted and perhaps definitive of these analyses. Kirsch's meta-analysis included all the major clinical trials of SSRI antidepressants—both those that were published and the nearly 40% that were withheld from publication by the pharmaceutical companies who sponsored or conducted them (the withheld trials largely showed negative results). Kirsch's analysis revealed the vast majority of people who took the antidepressant experienced, on average, no clinically significant improvement over those who took the placebo. "Antidepressants are supposed to work by fixing a chemical imbalance, specifically, a lack of serotonin in the brain. Indeed, their supposed effectiveness is the primary evidence for the chemical imbalance theory. But analyses of the published data and the unpublished data that were hidden by drug companies reveals that most (if not all) of the benefits are due to the placebo effect. Some antidepressants increase serotonin levels, some decrease it, and some have no effect at all on serotonin. Nevertheless, they all show the same therapeutic benefit. Even the small statistical difference between antidepressants and placebos may be an enhanced placebo effect, due to the fact that most patients and doctors in clinical trials successfully break blind. The serotonin theory is as close as any theory in the history of science to having been proved wrong."[44]

4
MENTAL HEALTH: THE BUSINESS

Treating our 'mental health' is big business. The more people diagnosed the more drugs are sold. But who is looking after the patients' interests?

If we see our ability to cope with life as an illness or condition, the drug regulators and pharmaceutical industry see us as customers. Antidepressants and other medications used in mental health have become a multi-billion-dollar business. What most of us don't realize is the regulators of antidepressants and other psychiatric drugs; the Federal Drug Agency (FDA) in the US and the Medicines and Healthcare products Regulatory Agency (MHRA) in the UK, receive significant funding from the pharmaceutical industry and employ ex-industry professionals in key leadership positions.[19]

The FDA is often accused of not putting the American people first. Little surprise when we look at the donations made to Senate members and the House of Representatives. During the 2017–2018 election campaigns, pharmaceutical companies donated $6,955,960 to Senate members and $16,823,447 to House of Representative members.[20] There is little doubt that the financial ties between pharma and congress are negatively affecting the health of the US by promoting our ongoing exposure to sometimes harmful prescription drugs. But this issue is also about a lack of consumer awareness. The pharmaceutical industry relies on us trusting them and that we choose to take their drugs. We need to be more aware and try to educate ourselves as best we can. We need to be in a position where we can make better, more informed decisions.

In the UK, the MHRA has often been accused of corruption. The costs it incurs for regulating medicines in the UK are, as the MHRA states, entirely "met by fees from the pharmaceutical industry". In other words, the regulation of all medical drugs in the UK (psychiatric and otherwise), is entirely funded by the very industry whose success or failure and most importantly profits, depend upon whether its products are approved by organizations like the MHRA.[21]

These conflicts of interest have been said to lead to lenient regulations placing commercial (pharmaceutical) interests above patient protection. Most of us will be surprised to hear the FDA and the MHRA require only two positive clinical trials to approve an antidepressant for public use. Without any clear scientific justification or rationale, the FDA and MHRA simply ignore the negative trials. This industry has a long history of burying negative results, and of manipulating research to highlight positive outcomes. The majority of psychiatric drug trials are of course conducted and commissioned by the pharmaceutical industry.

"The MHRA requires only 2 clinical trials to approve a psychiatric drug for public use, even if there exist 4, 5, 6, or more negative trials. In a practice for which there is no clear scientific justification or rationale, the MHRA simply discards the negative trials. This means, in short, that even if 10 negative trials exist, on the basis of only one or two positive trials the drug can still be approved for public use."[22]

In the UK, The House of Commons Health Committee has in the past criticized the process by which drugs are licensed, saying it is far from transparent. Their concerns include the facts there is no public access to the data presented by the pharmaceutical companies nor to the assessments undertaken by the MHRA. They say there is not enough involvement of patients, the public and the wider scientific community, the agency does not listen or communicate well and denial of access to information held by the MHRA puts the interests of pharmaceutical companies ahead of those of patients. "There is evidence that in certain areas, company influence is excessive and contrary to the public good. A distortion in the balance between industry and public interests can be seen as inappropriate not by breaching any law but because the very excess might be a destabilizing influence and put patients at risk."[23]

The latest FDA controversy came in March 2019, when they approved the antidepressant esketamine, to be marketed under the brand name Spravato, for treatment-resistant major depression. The FDA gave the pharmaceutical company Janssen very quick approval for Spravato and, it is reported, quite a bit of flexibility. Spravato, like the ketamine on which it is based, can have psychedelic and cognitive adverse effects. The nasal spray can only be administered in a medical setting and patients must stay at the clinic for at least two hours after administration.[24]

In Lancet Psychiatry online, Erick H. Turner, MD, who is a member of one of the FDA advisory committees which recommended approval of Spravato said, "the drug did not meet standard criteria for FDA approval and there was little evidence to support its safety and efficacy based on data from three short-term phase 3 trials and one withdrawal trial." Turner, who is a psychiatrist at Oregon Health and Science University in Portland, noted, "only one of the three trials that led to the drug's approval was positive, and there was a widespread assumption that a "breakthrough" drug with a novel mechanism of action is more effective than approved alternatives." He calls this "breakthrough bias." He added, "If you showed them the same data for an SSRI, they would ask, "What's good about this?"[25]

Another expert, Glen Spielmans, PhD, professor of psychology and antidepressant researcher, Metropolitan State University, Minnesota, told Medscape Medical News, "Based on the evidence provided in Janssen's application, the FDA should not have approved the drug. The fact that esketamine was superior to placebo to a statistically significant extent in only one of the short-term trials is unimpressive."[26]

What is worrying about this is by lowering the bar and approving antidepressants "with incredibly questionable safety and efficacy," the FDA is once again putting patients at risk. Any new antidepressants, from now on, may or may not "meet standard criteria for FDA approval" and yet they might still be approved! Time will tell, but this might prove to be just one more example of the FDA not putting the American people first.

Again, **this book does not contain medical advice**. Use this book to understand what antidepressants are and their possible benefits and risks, which include the many "side"/adverse effects. It is important to remember there is a real chance we might become dependent on antidepressants.

WARNING: There are many reasons why it is important we never stop taking or start withdrawing from antidepressants or other psychotropic medication without the support of a knowledgeable medical professional or support service. Antidepressant treatment should be supported by frequent reviews. We need to be aware, from the very first pill we take, of any physical or psychological changes we experience and report them immediately to our prescriber. Evidence suggests the risk of suicide, self-harm or other severe adverse events is significantly higher when commencing, stopping or changing doses or switching drugs including generics.

PART 2

The Power of the Informed Patient

5

ALTERNATIVES WORTH CONSIDERING

Life can be difficult, but the question is: Might our situation change? Might we simply feel better with time?

We have all become used to our ability to cope with our life being regarded as our "mental health". The reality is, we are, most of the time simply being human and reacting to everyday life events the way we as humans might be expected to. It is natural to be sad after a death, feel lost after a relationship breakup, anxious when we lose our job or feel traumatized after a major adverse experience. It is often difficult and painful but our emotions and reactions to our life are what make us who we are.

If we are finding life difficult to cope with, we might decide to visit a doctor or psychiatrist. If they are sensible and realistic, they might ask us to wait a while before we consider taking medication.[45] It would probably be worth taking their advice. A lot of the time we will start to feel better if we wait, even if to us it seems like the more difficult option. Life can be fast moving, ever changing, and the way we are feeling is probably a reaction to an aspect of our present life, however painful it might be. Former psychiatrist Dean Schuyler wrote in his 1974 book that most depressive episodes "will run their course and terminate with virtually complete recovery without specific intervention."[46]

Nowadays we are all told to be more open about our mental health. We are encouraged by governments, charities and celebrities to tell our "stories" about our mental state. The media bombard us with messages that our mental health is no different to our physical health; that they deserve parity, and we deserve help.

If we think about it rationally, we can often work out the real issues in our lives causing our sadness, anxiety, grief or distress. With the right support and a little time our feelings and life events, traumas, stresses and worries will probably pass, and we will learn from our experience. Life's ups and downs make us who we are and help us build our character. A lot of the time these events strengthen our ability to respond to future life events, however challenging they might be.

In 2006, Michael Posternak, a psychiatrist at Brown University studied what untreated major depression might look like today. His findings showed that old epidemiological studies were not so inaccurate at all and considered why six-week trials of drugs had been misleading. He reported that 22% of non-medicated patients recovered after one month; 67% within six months; and 85% within a year. He wrote, "If as many as 85% of depressed individuals who go without somatic treatment spontaneously recover within one year, it would be extremely difficult for any intervention to demonstrate a superior result to this."[47,48]

When we are finding life tough, we might consider asking for help but that doesn't always have to be professional help. We could talk to family, friends or a work colleague about how we feel about our life. We can share as much or as little as we need to. Most importantly we can ask them to listen to how we are feeling without them being judgmental or offering advice. This is not a conversation about our "mental health" but one about our life and things we might be struggling with or finding difficult. It is a great place to start.

Not everyone has someone to talk with or wants to share their feelings with people they know. We could ask to be referred for psychological therapy or counselling. It might not feel "like me" to ask for this kind of help but we might be surprised how much it can help us deal with the underlying causes of our emotional distress. The reality is it probably won't change the life situation we find our self in, but it might help us look at and cope with things differently.

There are many alternatives to consider before we turn to medication. Lifestyle improvements including our diet, sleep, drinking less alcohol and reducing screen time (in particular the time we spend on social media), can all have a positive effect on how we feel. Increasing exercise has proven positive benefits on our mental state. Spending time reading, gardening, with a pet, or taking up a new hobby can be effective ways to deal with anxiety or low mood. Everyone's situation is different, and we have to acknowledge not everyone is in a situation where we can turn to these alternatives. But it is important to remember that a life without antidepressants is an option and life well worth considering.

6
BEING INFORMED ABOUT OUR TREATMENT OPTIONS

It is about being as informed as we can be and asking about our treatment options.

The Nation Institute for Mental Health (NIMH) advise; "Treatment for mental illnesses usually consists of therapy, medication or a combination of the two. Treatment can be given in person or through a phone or computer (telehealth). It can sometimes be difficult to know where to start when looking for mental health care, but there are many ways to find a provider who will meet your needs."[49]

For low level depression, guidelines suggest an initial course of psychosocial therapy like guided self-help or physical activity and for low level to moderate depression, a high-intensity psychological therapy is recommended. If we are experiencing moderate to severe depression, guidance indicates antidepressants can be prescribed with a high-intensity psychological therapy. Guidance also suggests antidepressants can be used for people with low level to moderate depression if psychosocial and psychological treatments have not worked.

The suggestion is we should already have received psychological therapy or have been referred for psychological therapy prior to antidepressants being prescribed. The reality is there are many reasons we might not be offered therapy. Unfortunately, a large percentage of us have no access to psychosocial support or psychological therapy as services to refer people to often don't exist or have long waiting times.

Antidepressants are all too readily used as first-line treatment, with no other options discussed.

It is not easy, but we should always try to be as involved as we can be in planning and making decisions about our health care. When discussing treatment, it is important we make decisions with our doctor and that they listen to our opinions. Doctors should not make decisions about our treatment without asking how we feel and without informing us of our treatment options and their benefits and risks. It is important to remember we have the right to ask questions.

We need to be as prepared as we can be before attending an appointment. Having our views respected and having the opportunity and time to make a decision is our right and we owe it to ourselves to be as informed as we can be. If we make choices about our own treatment, we are more likely to benefit from it. Many of us do not want to take antidepressants, but we do know we need some kind of help. Our doctor should always give us the information and advice to enable us to get the best and most appropriate treatment available.

Using this book and being more informed about antidepressants can make us feel more confident about being involved in making decisions about our treatment. Where possible we should try to include our family or someone close to us when we are thinking about taking antidepressants. We can often have symptoms which might prevent us making fully informed decisions and, if this is the case, it is important to take someone with us to appointments and have their support. They can ask questions on our behalf and try to get honest answers. We do not have to make a decision about antidepressants at our first appointment or even immediately after receiving a prescription. We could take some time, use this book to help with our decision, talk to others who have experience of taking them, weigh up our options and decide what is best for us.

7
THE IMPORTANCE OF INFORMED CONSENT

Are we being fully informed when we are prescribed antidepressants? Why does this area of medicine seem to ignore "informed consent"?

In nearly all other areas of medicine (such as surgery, medical tests and procedures), a patient's informed consent is required prior to treatment. This means a prescriber must explain the treatment so that we can decide if the treatment is right for us. We should be in a position where we can make educated decisions and informed choices, with our prescriber, about what is best for us. *Informed consent means we understand why, based on our diagnosis, the treatment is being offered and we are aware of the benefits and risks.* Only then should we agree to the treatment. Informed consent is our medical right.

Rather than informed consent, antidepressant prescribing has sometimes been described as being based on "manufactured consent". This implies we are being manipulated into supporting what others want us to support but we believe we are forming our opinion using our own free will. Whether it be "manufactured" or "implied" consent, anything other than informed consent is unacceptable when being prescribed mind-altering antidepressants.

"Why has the American public not heard psychiatrists in positions of influence on the mass media debunking the chemical imbalance theory? Big Pharma's corruption of psychiatry is only part of the explanation. Many psychiatrists, acting in the manner of a benevolent elite, did not alert the general public because they believed that the chemical imbalance theory was a useful fiction to get patients to accept their mental illness and take their medication. In other words, the chemical imbalance theory was an excellent way to manufacture consent."[50]

Wendy Ratcliffe and Lynn Cunningham, directors of the documentary, "Medicating Normal,"[51] a film showing the experiences of people harmed by taking psychiatric medication, want psychiatrists and doctors to require informed consent for all psychiatric drug prescriptions. "The problem, Ratcliffe says, is that psychiatry lobbying groups feel that informed consent impedes their ability to prescribe. She compares the industry to the NRA: any criticism is treated as a potential keystone that, if removed, will take out the entire system. In reality, all patients are asking for is honesty about how these drugs interact in their bodies. We don't know the long-term effects because pharmaceutical companies don't have to study them. If the industry isn't required to disclose these effects, and psychiatrists remain ignorant of the real damage being done to some of their patients, informed consent remains an intangible dream with no pathway to reality."[52]

A 2012 University of Massachusetts Boston study concluded, "Clinicians today practice in a time-limited, pharmaceutical-industry dominated climate in which reductive biological models are heavily promoted. Such models reinforce an acontextual view of patients' problems and a disease- rather than patient-centered model of care. As a result, "diagnosis by checklist" (Andreasen, 2007) becomes a primary source of automatic prescribing (Cosgrove & Bursztajn, 2007). Thus, genuine informed consent requires, first and foremost, that mental health professionals adopt a mindful approach to psychiatric taxonomy and be aware not only of the uses, but also the limitations of and alternatives to psychopharmacological interventions. Respecting patient autonomy requires that clinicians be aware of the marketing practices and biases that may distort their appraisal of the relative risks and benefits of medications such as antidepressants, and moreover that they consider the ways in which people can be manipulated by social constructions of normalcy and health in an industry-dominated climate (see e.g., Ells, 2003). This increasingly complex network of considerations presents distinct challenges for clinicians, but dynamic informed consent processes offer a way to acknowledge the uncertainty associated with antidepressants while simultaneously empowering patients in their recovery from illness."

To enable informed consent, doctors would have to confront some uncomfortable issues which include many of the questionable beliefs on which their prescribing is based; the unproven chemical imbalance theory, the huge risks, the lack of scientific evidence. They would have to explain to us that we might find we are taking antidepressants in the long term, that there is a lack of evidence to support this practice and there are no protocols to help us withdraw if we become dependent.

"Given the drug commercial propaganda onslaught, for the American people to become aware of the truth, psychiatrists in positions of influence would have had to zealously publicize that the research had rejected the chemical imbalance theory, and they would have had to use the mass media to proclaim that the drug commercials are false."[53]

Requiring informed consent when prescribing antidepressants would undoubtedly change prescribing habits. Informed consent would also mean we need answers to the many questions about the evidence on which antidepressants are currently prescribed. Some doctors do make sure their patients are fully informed, but for the foreseeable future at least, the best we can do is educate ourselves and those we care about.

In our quick fix world, three minutes is all it might take to be diagnosed "mentally ill".

Millions have been diagnosed as having depression or anxiety using the questionnaires PHQ-9 and GAD-7. These were designed to enable doctors to recognize depression disorders and anxiety disorders. Adopted as standard measures, these screening tools set a very low threshold for what can be diagnosed as mental illness according to DSM criteria. They can take less than three minutes to complete. Our responses to these questions often result in a pharmaceutical company's questionnaire and a doctor's subjective decision determining whether or not we are mentally ill and which treatment and label we receive.

The copyright for the PHQ-9 was formerly held with Pfizer Pharmaceuticals. They provided the educational grant for the design of the questionnaire. They no longer hold the copyright and no permission is required to reproduce, translate, display or distribute the PHQ-9. Of course, the more doctors use the questionnaires, the more antidepressants and other psychotropic drugs are sold. Pfizer are the makers of the SSRI antidepressant Zoloft (sertraline), the SNRI antidepressant Effexor (venlafaxine).

PHQ-9[54]				
Over the last 2 weeks, how often have you been bothered by any of the following problems?:	**Not at all**	**Several days**	**More than half the days**	**Nearly every day**
1. Little interest or pleasure in doing things	0	1	2	3
2. Feeling down, depressed, or hopeless	0	1	2	3
3. Trouble falling or staying asleep, or sleeping too much	0	1	2	3
4. Feeling tired or having little energy	0	1	2	3
5. Poor appetite or overeating	0	1	2	3
6. Feeling bad about yourself—or that you are a failure or have let yourself or your family down	0	1	2	3
7. Trouble concentrating on things, such as reading the newspaper or watching television	0	1	2	3
8. Moving or speaking so slowly that other people could have noticed? Or the opposite—being so fidgety or restless that you have been moving around a lot more than usual	0	1	2	3
9. Thoughts that you would be better off dead or of hurting yourself in some way	0	1	2	3
	add columns:	______ +	______ +	______

PHQ-9 TOTAL SCORE = ☐

If you checked off any problems above, how difficult have these problems made it for you to do your work, take care of things at home, or get along with other people?

Not difficult at all	Somewhat difficult	Very difficult	Extremely difficult
☐	☐	☐	☐

GAD-7[54]				
Over the last 2 weeks, how often have you been bothered by any of the following problems?:	**Not at all**	**Several days**	**More than half the days**	**Nearly every day**
1. Feeling nervous, anxious, or on edge	0	1	2	3
2. Not being able to stop or control worrying	0	1	2	3
3. Worrying too much about different things	0	1	2	3
4. Trouble relaxing	0	1	2	3
5. Being so restless that it is hard to sit still	0	1	2	3
6. Becoming easily annoyed or irritable	0	1	2	3
7. Feeling afraid as if something awful might happen	0	1	2	3
	add columns:	______ +	______ +	______

GAD-7 TOTAL SCORE= ☐

If you checked off any problems above, how difficult have these problems made it for you to do your work, take care of things at home, or get along with other people?

Not difficult at all	Somewhat difficult	Very difficult	Extremely difficult
☐	☐	☐	☐

PHQ-9 Score	GAD-7 Score	Severity	Proposed Treatment Actions
0–4	0–5	None	None
5–9	6–10	Mild	Watchful waiting, repeating at follow-up.
10–14	11–15	Moderate	Consider CBT and pharmacotherapy
15–19	—	Moderately Severe	Initiation of pharmacotherapy and CBT.
20–27	16–21	Severe	Initiation of pharmacotherapy and CBT. Consider specialist referral to psychiatrist.

8
KNOWING ANTIDEPRESSANT BENEFITS AND RISKS

If we are thinking about taking antidepressants, we need to look at the benefits and risks. We need to be aware of the lack of scientific evidence on which antidepressant prescribing is based.

It is important to remember that antidepressants can be prescribed for a wide range of problems. They are used to treat anxiety, insomnia, pain, smoking cessation, premenstrual syndrome, panic disorders, fibromyalgia, migraine, obsessive-compulsive disorders, and a host of other "off-label" conditions for which the drugs are not even approved.

Since they were introduced, the benefits of antidepressants have been widely promoted and the risks generally downplayed. We read so many times that if we have been diagnosed and prescribed antidepressants, "it's just like taking medicine for a physical condition" and they are simply "another treatment option to help you get better." This is grossly oversimplified and is in many cases untrue.

Everyone has an individual, unique response to antidepressants and even though there are some very common experiences when first starting to take them, no one can predict how we will react to them physically and psychologically. During the first few weeks some of the adverse effects we might experience are: nausea, insomnia, increased anxiety, restlessness, dizziness, weight gain, dry mouth, sweating, upset stomach, headaches, agitation, loss of appetite and decreased sex drive, amongst others.

A doctor should always give us comprehensive information when prescribing antidepressants allowing for fully informed decision making. We might be told "antidepressants take four to six weeks to work." We also often hear, "It is completely normal for antidepressants to make you feel worse before you feel better" and that our bodies and minds are "adjusting to a new medication". But are we adjusting to the drugs or, as Stephen Hyman wrote, are antidepressants making changes to our brains and how we function?[55] Are the changes the first signs of dependence and the beginning of our new "antidepressed" drug-induced normal?

If we have unpleasant side or adverse effects after the first two weeks, we might go back to our prescriber. We might be switched from one antidepressant to another until we find the one that best suits us. We might be told that finding the right antidepressant is a process of trial and error, but it might simply be that eventually the antidepressants create our new "qualitatively and quantitatively different" balanced state. We simply don't know. We are told "the efficacy of the different antidepressants is largely equivalent," so perhaps we might trust our doctor to find us the one which has the least adverse effects until we get used to these changes?

Actual positive response rates to antidepressants are much lower in studies with "real-world" patients compared to industry-funded trials. In a study of 118 real-world outpatients, only 19% of the patients had responded to an antidepressant after three months, which is a much lower response rate than is usually seen in the industry-funded trials. The NIMH funded a large study, known as the STAR*D study, to assess the effectiveness of antidepressants in real-world patients, and even though patients were given up to four courses of treatment with different antidepressants, only 38% ever responded positively to the treatment.[56]

It is important to note the Patient Information Leaflets accompanying antidepressants state, "the side effects depend on the dose and often disappear or lessen with continued treatment"; the pharmaceutical companies would of course prefer we continue taking our medication.

Adverse effects might lessen or disappear simply because we get used to the drug's actions and the changes, but it could be at the expense of many aspects of our life and health being detrimentally affected. The most significant being becoming dependent on the medication.

After a few weeks of taking antidepressants many of us decide they are not for us and look for other ways to help. For others it can seem like antidepressants have been lifesaving and it can become difficult to imagine surviving without them. The reality might be that with or without the medication, things in our life might simply have changed, improved, moved on, got better and in the meantime, we have started a life where "difficulty surviving without antidepressants" has actually become a physical and psychological reality.

> If we choose to start taking antidepressants, we must have frequent reviews with our prescriber. If we choose to take an antidepressant, we must be aware of any physical and psychological changes. At any time during treatment, we need to note these and report them to our prescriber. It is our right to ask questions and be an informed patient. Having thoughts of suicide, self-harm or violence are linked to starting antidepressant treatment. In 2004, the US Food and Drug Administration, (FDA) issued a black box warning—the agency's strictest warning—for all SSRI antidepressants regarding their association with suicidal thoughts and behaviors. It is for this reason it is vital, if possible, we let someone close to us know if we start taking antidepressants. They can monitor any changes in our behavior and personality which we might not recognize ourselves. Any changes should be immediately reported to our prescriber.

A doctor or psychiatrist should give us comprehensive information when prescribing antidepressants enabling us to make fully informed decisions. Unfortunately, we know this does not always happen.

According to Realistic Medicine in the UK, one of the ways forward is "Choosing Wisely", a set of question prompts which some National Health Service (NHS) Scotland boards are encouraging people to ask about their health care.

1. Is this test, treatment or procedure really needed?
2. What are the potential benefits and risks?
3. What are the possible side effects?
4. Are there simpler, safer or alternative treatment options?
5. What would happen if I did nothing?[57]

Preparing for an appointment with our doctor:

- Before going to an appointment, we should think about and write down any questions we have.
- Write down our symptoms, how we are feeling and our main concerns. Try to remember how long we have had any symptoms, their severity and how they have changed over time.
- Take a list of any medications we are currently taking, including both prescription and over-the-counter medications and any supplements /vitamins. This should include the dose and how often we take them.
- During the appointment take notes we can refer back to later.
- It is particularly important to discuss any psychological therapy / counselling we have had or antidepressants we have taken in the past.
- Take a note of any other medical conditions we have.
- If we do not feel confident or comfortable asking questions, it might be useful to ask a relative or friend to go with us to our appointment. Tell them how we are feeling before the appointment and the questions we need to ask.

Some questions we might want to ask about our treatment:

- Why do you think I am feeling the way I am?
- Why do you think I should take antidepressants and what are their benefits?
- Are there other options to antidepressants-such as 'social prescribing' and/or psychotherapy/counselling -and can you give me information on what is available to me?
- If I decide to take an antidepressant, which would you prescribe and why?
- Is this antidepressant approved to help me?
- How would I take the medication?
- What happens if I were to miss a dose?
- What are the adverse effects and what should I do if I have any?
- How soon will the antidepressants work?
- What do I need to avoid while on this medication?
- How long will I need to be on this medication?
- Can I become addicted to or dependent on antidepressants?
- Can I stop taking this medication when I feel better?
- Will I get help when I decide to stop taking them?
- What should I be doing in addition to taking medication?
- Should I let a relative or friend know I have started this medication?
- Antidepressant prescribing is based on scientific evidence… isn't it?

The American Psychiatric Association's (APA) website Practice Guidelines says they "provide evidence-based recommendations for the assessment and treatment of psychiatric disorders." They claim their guidelines are evidence-based practice but actually have only three current and up-to-date guidelines available.

"The APA developed and published 23 practice guidelines from 1992 to 2010, including multiple second and third editions. Thirteen of the guidelines are available in this section. These guidelines are more than 5 years old and have not yet been updated to ensure that they reflect current knowledge and practice. In accordance with national standards, including those of the Agency for Healthcare Research and Quality's National Guideline Clearinghouse, these guidelines can no longer be assumed to be current."[58]

Prescribing is the area most affected by evidence-based medicine, "the conscientious, explicit, and judicious use of current best evidence in making decisions about the care of individual patients."[59] Few other areas of medical practice have felt the effects of this movement more than prescribing of medicines. If governments and medical bodies claim they are implementing evidence-based prescribing for antidepressants then they should be expected to back up their decisions with evidence and this should rely on honest data, clinical expertise and patients' values and preferences. All this should result in the safer and more effective use of antidepressants.

The UK Royal College of Psychiatrists 2019 position statement on antidepressants and depression states, "It is worth noting that a challenge in prescribing antidepressants is that the available research does not inform clinicians about whether an individual patient will benefit from antidepressant use, to what extent, and which type of antidepressant should be tried first. Clinicians therefore need to use their judgement, training, and experience in discussing and agreeing the best approach with patients and/or their family/care providers."[60]

Unfortunately, it is all too apparent that, based on the current evidence available, the claims that antidepressants and other drugs used in mental health work and are safe is very questionable. There have been only a few other medications that have had such large numbers of double-blinded, placebo-controlled trials performed to demonstrate they work and gain regulatory approval. There have been over a thousand antidepressant randomized trials and statistically significant benefits have been repeatedly demonstrated. The medical profession and patients found this evidence reassuring and few questions were asked.

Despite all of this, the truth is unfavorable trials are frequently left unpublished and remain unavailable to doctors and patients. This is a process of selective publication and study-designs are often manipulated and industry-sponsored studies are incomplete, biased and in favor of their product. It is a fact that most intervention studies are industry sponsored. The medical profession and the public are often being misled, and this means patients can be given less effective, harmful or more expensive treatments.

Contrary to what we have been told and what most of us believe, the genuine antidepressant "evidence-based" facts include:

- There are no known biological causes for any of the mental health disorders apart from dementia and some rare chromosomal disorders.
- Mental health diagnostic systems lack validity.
- No chemical imbalances have been proven to exist in relation to any mental health disorder.
- Antidepressants do not 'cure' diseases, and in many cases their mechanism of action is not properly understood.
- Psychiatric drugs cause altered mental states.
- Studies have found that antidepressants have no clinically significant benefits over placebo pills in the treatment of mild to moderate depression.
- Negative effects are often misdiagnosed.
- There has been little research on the long-term outcomes of people taking antidepressants and they can have effects including mental disturbance, suicide, violence, and withdrawal syndromes.
- The majority of psychiatric drug trials are conducted and commissioned by the pharmaceutical industry or those who have extensive ties with them. This industry has a long history of burying negative results, and of manipulating research to highlight positive outcomes.
- Withdrawal from antidepressants can be disabling and cause severe physical and psychological effects which often last for months and sometimes years, sometimes leading to suicide.

More information on these facts can be found at "Unrecognized Facts" published by the UK Council for Evidence-Based Psychiatry.[61]

Off-label prescribing...when there is no evidence at all!

We might be surprised to learn a large percentage of antidepressants are prescribed off-label. Off-label prescribing is when an FDA-approved medication is prescribed for an unapproved condition or in different way from that approved by the FDA. The prescribing of medications in this manner is definitely not supported by scientific evidence.

"From the FDA perspective, once the FDA approves a drug, healthcare providers generally may prescribe the drug for an unapproved use when they judge that it is medically appropriate for their patient. You may be asking yourself why your healthcare provider would want to prescribe a drug to treat a disease or medical condition that the drug is not approved for. One reason is that there might not be an approved drug to treat your disease or medical condition. Another is that you may have tried all approved treatments without seeing any benefits. In situations like these, you and your healthcare provider may talk about using an approved drug for an unapproved use to treat your disease or medical condition."[62]

Investigators at McGill University, in Montreal, Canada, found that 45% of the antidepressants prescribed for more than 100,000 adults living in the province of Quebec were for conditions other than depression. Furthermore, almost one third of these prescriptions were for an off-label indication, most commonly, insomnia and pain. "Researchers want to assess the safety and effectiveness of different antidepressants, but one of the main problems standing in the way of that is that physicians are prescribing antidepressants for so many different indications now, not just depression."[63] "The off-label use of prescription drugs was associated with a 44% increase in the risk of adverse drug events and an even greater risk, 54%, when the off-label use was not backed by strong scientific evidence. Off-label prescribing is common, with one US study finding that about a fifth of doctors' prescriptions were for off-label use."[64]

There is an urgent need to produce more evidence of the risks and benefits of off-label antidepressant use and a need for improved monitoring and evaluating of off-label use. Off-label prescribing can put us at risk of adverse effects and unknown health risks which could be avoided. Of particular concern is the growing rate of off-label prescribing of antidepressants to children and young adults. As patients we need to know if we are being prescribed antidepressants off-label and we should always ask the question, "Is this medication approved to treat my condition?" It is important we ask why we are being prescribed antidepressants if they have not been approved to treat us. It is just one more area of antidepressant prescribing where we can be at the mercy of the subjective "medical judgement" and the scientifically unfounded opinion of our doctor.

9
THE MANY ADVERSE EFFECTS INCLUDING AKATHISIA

Antidepressants might have no clinically significant benefit over placebos, but these licensed and widely prescribed medications can cause serious adverse effects.

It is misguided to believe the "placebo effect" is justification for taking antidepressants. Rather than being inert, we know they can induce varied and unpredictable physical and mental states.[65] They are not a cure for any mental health condition, and the adverse effects of these drugs can be serious and sometimes even fatal, making the description of these drugs as "working at placebo-level" misleading and unrealistic. Antidepressants disrupt the function of key neurotransmitters which play important roles throughout the main communications systems of both our brain and body, a fact often ignored or denied by prescribers.

"The public is being misinformed about the precision of these selective serotonin-uptake inhibitors when the medical profession oversimplifies their action in the brain and ignores the body as if it exists merely to carry the head around! In short, these molecules of emotion regulate every aspect of our physiology."[66]

In some cases, antidepressants can create health problems we did not have prior to taking the medication and their benefits are limited. Recent research and the ever-growing body of anecdotal evidence confirms the seriousness of antidepressant adverse effects. It is impossible to list every adverse effect we might suffer when taking an antidepressant. How they affect us as an individual is unique to us. For some, adverse effects can happen at recommended dose levels and when taken short term, and for others it can be dependent on the dose or on which antidepressant we are prescribed.

Common adverse effects of antidepressants include central nervous system problems, sexual problems, weight gain, digestive problems, debilitating fatigue and numbed emotions, as well as other confusing and little understood symptoms. It is now blatantly obvious these so called "side effects" contribute significantly to other health, relationship, social and economic issues, and increasingly to the national burden of chronic ill-health and disability rates.

A 2018 study concluded, "Asking people directly reveals far higher rates of adverse responses to antidepressants than previously understood, especially in the emotional, psychological and interpersonal domains. Given recent findings that antidepressants are only marginally more effective than placebo, the findings of the current study imply a cost-benefit analysis that cannot justify the extremely high prescription rates for these drugs."[67] The online survey asked antidepressant users whether they had experienced 20 adverse effects and to what degree of severity. The survey included 1,431 people, from 38 countries.[68]

PERCENTAGES OF 1,431 ANTIDEPRESSANT USERS WHO REPORTED EACH ADVERSE EFFECT	
Feeling emotionally numb	70.6%
Feeling foggy or detached	70.0%
Feeling not like myself	66.2%
Sexual difficulties	66.1%
Drowsiness	62.7%
Reduction in positive feelings	60.4%
Weight gain	60.1%
Dry mouth	59.3%
Distorted dreams	59.2%
Withdrawal effects	58.9%

PERCENTAGES OF 1,431 ANTIDEPRESSANT USERS WHO REPORTED EACH ADVERSE EFFECT	
Agitation	58.0%
Insomnia	57.7%
Caring less about others	54.5%
Dizziness	51.6%
Headaches	50.4%
Suicidality	50.3%

Doctors are prescribing these powerful drugs as "safe and effective", but they can have complex neurological effects some prescribers do not seem to want to understand or acknowledge. When we report symptoms, we can often be disbelieved and discounted by doctors. We can also fail to realize ourselves that it is our medication, "taken as prescribed", which is causing the symptoms we are experiencing. It is common for doctors to add more medications to deal with what are antidepressant adverse effects. This can result in polypharmacy and further complications.

It is crucial we recognize any changes we experience when taking antidepressants, particularly when starting, withdrawing from them or changing dose. Any adverse effects or changes must be reported to our prescriber. It is important we ask the question "could my antidepressant be causing my problems?" and we do not simply assume our doctor knows all the side /adverse effects of the drugs we take.

In the Washington Post article, "Doctors often don't tell you about drug side effects, and that's a problem," Adriane Fugh-Berman, professor in the Department of Pharmacology and Physiology at Georgetown University Medical Center says, "Patients need to become their own experts, researching drugs on websites—such as the government database

MedlinePlus[69,70]—that are free of [the pharmaceutical] industry. Doctors have a responsibility to listen to their patients about side effects, too, she said. I tell medical students: If a patient develops a symptom after they've gone on their drug, it's always the drug's fault until proven otherwise. We're in sort of a bad situation now where the people in control of prescribing drugs know the least about the drugs."[71]

So that we can provide informed consent, our doctors should inform us of the possible adverse effects before we agree to take antidepressants. But to protect ourselves, we need to ask questions. We need to ask ourselves, do antidepressants balance a non-existent chemical brain imbalance or is there the potential they might actually create disturbing brain and body imbalances? We need to be aware the harmful and life-changing adverse effects of antidepressants experienced by some patients point to the latter.

Some of the more common "adverse" or "side" effects of antidepressants include:

- Gastrointestinal effects, such as nausea, diarrhea, dyspepsia, GI bleeding and abdominal pain
- Hepatotoxicity and hypersensitivity reactions; liver toxicity, fever and rash
- Weight problems and metabolic disturbances; weight gain, anorexia
- Cardiovascular effects, such as heart rate variability leading to cardiovascular events
- Genitourinary ailments like urinary retention, incontinence
- Sexual dysfunction, reductions in libido, arousal dysfunction
- Hyponatremia; salt imbalance
- Osteoporosis/bone weakening, risk of fractures, loss of muscle strength fatigue
- Abnormal bleeding and bruising

- Nervous system dysfunction: akathisia followed by dystonic reactions, parkinsonian movements and tardive dyskinesia, headaches, tremors, numbness, tingling, burning
- Sweating
- Sleep disturbances: somnolence or sleepiness/insomnia
- Affective disturbances; mood change, emotional blunting, anxiety, agitation, panic attacks, insomnia, irritability, hostility, aggressiveness insomnia, impulsivity
- Overdose toxicity
- Withdrawal Syndrome: flu-like symptoms, tremors, tachycardia, shock-like sensations, paresthesia, myalgia, tinnitus, neuralgia, ataxia, vertigo, sexual dysfunction, sleep disturbances, vivid dreams, nausea, vomiting, diarrhea, worsening anxiety and mood instability, mania, psychosis
- Ophthalmic effects: glaucoma, cataracts, blurred/double vision
- Hyperprolactinemia; increases in peripheral prolactin levels
- Hormonal imbalance
- Risks during pregnancy and breast feeding, birth defects
- Risk of malignancies; growth of fibrosarcoma and melanoma
- Serotonin Syndrome
- Suicidality[72]

A Patient Information Leaflet (PIL) for sertraline (very similar to the PIL for other SSRI/SNRI antidepressants) lists over *fifty* possible "side effects" which they describe as very common or common. In addition, there are over one hundred and forty which they describe as uncommon or rare. It explains side effects "often disappear or lessen with continued treatment." It is now recognized it is misleading for "drug dependence" to be listed as a rare side effect.

PACKAGE LEAFLET: INFORMATION FOR THE USER

Sertraline 50 mg & 100 mg film-coated Tablets Sertraline hydrochloride[73]

Like all medicines, this medicine can cause side effects, although not everybody gets them. Nausea is the most common side effect. The side effects depend on the dose and often disappear or lessen with continued treatment.

Tell your doctor immediately if you experience any of the following symptoms after taking this medicine, these symptoms can be serious.

- If you develop a severe skin rash that causes blistering (erythema multiforme); this can affect the mouth and tongue. These may be signs of a condition known as Stevens Johnson Syndrome, or Toxic Epidermal Necrolysis (TEN).

Your doctor will stop treatment in these cases:

- Allergic reaction or allergy which may include symptoms such as itchy skin rash, breathing problems, wheezing, swollen eyelids, face or lips.
- If you experience agitation, confusion, diarrhea, high temperature and blood pressure, excessive sweating and rapid heartbeat. These are symptoms of Serotonin Syndrome. In rare cases this syndrome may occur when you are taking certain medicines at the same time as sertraline.
- Your doctor may wish to stop your treatment if you develop yellow skin and eyes which may mean liver damage.
- If you experience depressive symptoms with ideas of harming or killing yourself (suicidal thoughts).
- If you start to get feelings of restlessness and are not able to sit or stand still after you start to take Sertraline film-coated Tablets. You should tell your doctor if you start to feel restless.
- If you have a fit (seizure).
- If you have a manic episode (see section 2, "Warnings and precautions").

The following side effects were seen in clinical trials in adults and after marketing.

Very common (may affect more than 1 in 10 people):

- Insomnia
- Dizziness
- Sleepiness
- Headache

- Diarrhea
- Feeling sick
- Dry mouth
- Ejaculation failure
- Fatigue

Common (may affect up to 1 in 10 people):

- Chest cold, sore throat, runny nose
- Decreased appetite, increased appetite
- Anxiety, depression, agitation, decreased sexual interest, nervousness, feeling strange, nightmare, teeth grinding
- Shaking, muscular movement problems (such as moving a lot, tense muscles, difficulty walking and stiffness, spasms and involuntary movements of muscles), numbness and tingling, muscle tense, lack of attention, abnormal taste
- Visual disturbance, ringing in ears
- Palpitations, hot flush, yawning
- Upset stomach, constipation, abdominal pain, vomiting, gas
- Increased sweating, rash, back pain, joint pain, muscle pain
- Menstrual irregularities, erectile dysfunction
- Malaise, chest pain, weakness, fever
- Weight increases
- Injury

Uncommon (may affect up to 1 in 100 people):

- Gastroenteritis, ear infection
- Tumor
- Hypersensitivity, seasonal allergy
- Low thyroid hormones
- Suicidal thoughts, suicidal behavior*, psychotic disorder, thinking abnormal, lack of caring, hallucinations, aggression, euphoric mood, paranoia
- Amnesia, decreased feeling, involuntary muscle contractions, passing out, moving a lot, migraine, convulsion, dizziness while standing up, abnormal coordination, speech disorder

* *Side effect reported after marketing*

- Enlarged pupils, ear pain, fast heartbeat, heart problem
- Bleeding problems (such as stomach bleeding)*, high blood pressure, flushing, blood in urine
- Shortness of breath, nosebleed, breathing difficult, possible wheezing
- Tarry stools, tooth disorder, inflammation of the esophagus, tongue problem, hemorrhoids, increased saliva, difficulty swallowing, burping, tongue disorder
- Eye swelling, hives, hair loss, itching, purple spots on skin, skin problems with blisters, dry skin, face oedema, cold sweat
- Osteoarthritis, muscle twitching, muscle cramps*, muscular weakness
- Increase in frequency of urination, problem urinating, unable to urinate, urinary incontinence, increase in urination, nighttime urination
- Sexual dysfunction, excessive vaginal bleeding, vaginal hemorrhage female sexual dysfunction
- Swelling in legs, chills, difficulty walking, thirst
- Increase in liver enzyme levels, weight decreased
- Cases of suicidal ideation and suicidal behaviors have been reported during sertraline therapy or rarely after treatment discontinuation (see section 2).

Rare (may affect up to 1 in 1,000 people):

- Diverticulitis, swollen lymph glands, decrease in clotting cells*, decrease in white blood cells*
- High cholesterol, problems controlling blood sugar levels (diabetes), low blood sugar, increase in blood sugar levels*, low blood salt*
- Physical symptoms due to stress or emotions, terrifying abnormal dreams, drug dependence, sleep walking, premature ejaculation
- Coma, abnormal movements, difficulty moving, increased sensation, sudden severe headache (which may be a sign of a serious condition known as reversible cerebral vasoconstriction syndrome (rcvs))*, sensory disturbance
- Spots in front of the eyes, glaucoma, double vision, light hurts eye, blood in the eye, unequal sized pupils, vision abnormal*, tear problems
- Heart attack, light-headedness, fainting, or chest discomfort which could be signs of changes in the electrical activity (seen on electrocardiogram) or abnormal rhythm of the heart*, slow heartbeat

* *Side effect reported after marketing*

- Poor circulation of arms and legs
- Breathing fast, progressive scarring of lung tissue
- (interstitial lung disease)*, closing up of throat, difficulty talking, breathing slow, hiccups
- Mouth ulceration, pancreatitis*, blood in stool, tongue ulceration, sore mouth
- Problems with liver function, serious liver function problems*, yellow skin and eyes (jaundice)
- Skin reaction to sun*, skin oedema*, hair texture abnormal, skin odor abnormal, hair rash
- Breakdown of muscle tissue*, bone disorder
- Urinary hesitation, decreased urination
- Breast discharge, dry vaginal area, genital discharge, red painful penis and foreskin, breast enlargement, prolonged erection
- Hernia, drug tolerance decreased
- Increase in blood cholesterol levels, abnormal laboratory tests*, semen abnormal, problems with clotting*
- Relaxation of blood vessels procedure

Not known; i.e. frequency cannot be estimated from the available data:

- Lock jaw*
- Bedwetting*
- Partial loss of vision

Additional side effects in children and adolescents

In clinical trials with children and adolescents, the side effects were generally similar to adults (see above). The most common side effects in children and adolescents were headache, insomnia, diarrhea and feeling sick.

Symptoms that can occur when treatment is discontinued

If you suddenly stop taking this medicine you may experience side effects such as dizziness, numbness, sleep disturbances, agitation or anxiety, headaches, feeling sick, being sick and shaking (see section 3 "If you stop taking Sertraline film-coated Tablets").

An increased risk of bone fractures has been observed in patients taking this type of medicine.

* *Side effect reported after marketing*

RxISK has a side effect checker. It can be very useful to take the RxISK report to our prescriber and discuss any side effects we are experiencing.

Experiencing a Drug Side Effect? Get your free RxISK Report to find out at www.Rxisk.org

All prescription drugs can cause side effects, but it can often be difficult to engage with your doctor when your treatment might be causing a problem.

The RxISK Report takes 10 minutes to complete and provides you with a RxISK Score indicating how likely it is that your problem is caused by a prescription drug.

It can also help identify problems caused by stopping a drug—for example, withdrawal side effects.

If something is going wrong with your treatment, bringing a RxISK Report to your doctor as early as possible may be the difference between successful treatment and long-term disability or death.

No personally identifiable information is required—only your email address so that we can send you a printable PDF that you can take to your doctor.

The RxISK Report is designed to:

- Provide you with a RxISK Score to help determine whether your problem (or that of someone you care for) is linked to treatment.
- Inform and support a conversation with your doctor.
- Help our researchers improve drug safety with anonymized data.

"Akathisia": the one adverse effect of antidepressants we all need to be aware of.

"Akathisia is an extremely distressing neuropsychiatric syndrome characterized by severe agitation, inability to remain still, and an overwhelming sense of terror. It is primarily a medication side effect. People with this condition can quickly become suicidal and even homicidal. Akathisia is far more common than has been reported in the past and remains dangerously under-diagnosed and under-reported today."[75]

Akathisia is a medication-induced state and is mostly caused by antidepressants, antipsychotics, benzodiazepines, antibiotics, and anti-nausea medication. Akathisia is often described as the epitome of losing our mind, with our mind being taken over by uncontrollable and unrecognizable thoughts. It can happen when our minds become unbalanced due to starting, stopping or changing dose of certain medication or switching medication. It can cause terrifying symptoms, often confused with psychosis, which can also include intense physical restlessness and agitation often with a need for constant movement. It causes an inner turmoil with severe dysphoria (anxiety and agitation), manifesting as an overwhelming sense of terror. It can cause suicidal and violent impulses. Many people diagnosed with first episode psychosis are actually suffering from prescribed drug-induced akathisia.

"Akathisia is an emotional state caused by over 100 different drugs, primarily antidepressants and antipsychotics, but also antibiotics, anti-hypertensives and others. It causes suicidality, homicidality and other disturbances of behavior.[76] It can range from a constant and disturbing mental unease through to an intense emotional turmoil and mental restlessness. This can be accompanied by physical discomfort, an inability to remain still, or an obvious motor restlessness or fidgetiness. The problems caused by treatment can in many cases be worse than the illness being treated.[77] It may start within an hour of a first pill or only appear after days, weeks or months. It may only start when the dose of the drug is increased or decreased, or the drug is stopped. Akathisia is often misleadingly described as a movement disorder."

There are four types of akathisia. Each depends on when the problem occurs and how long it lasts:

- **Acute akathisia** develops shortly after starting a drug.
- **Tardive akathisia** develops months after starting the drug.
- **Withdrawal akathisia** occurs when stopping a drug.
- **Chronic akathisia** is any type that lasts for more than six months.[78]

Education and support for akathisia can be found online. It is vital we are made aware of and informed about akathisia when we are first prescribed our medication.[79] There is also an urgent need to educate the medical profession, social care workers and emergency services, so they can recognize and warn patients of the potential dangers of akathisia. Akathisia is a cause of both suicide and homicide, and it is time for governments, suicide prevention organizations and charities to recognize prescription drug-induced akathisia as a leading cause of suicide around the world.

Akathisia 101

MISSD is pleased to now offer Akathisia 101. The free, online one-hour continuing education course is open to all who want to better understand, identify and respond to akathisia. Akathisia 101 is approved by the National Association of Social Workers for 1 continuing education contact hour. Healthcare and crisis teams, patients, therapists, caregivers, doctors, first-responders, drug safety advocates and educators—everyone can benefit from akathisia awareness. Let's make Akathisia a household word (www.missd.co).

Akathisia Alliance for Education and Research

Akathisia Alliance for Education and Research has produced an invaluable Comprehensive Guide to Akathisia.

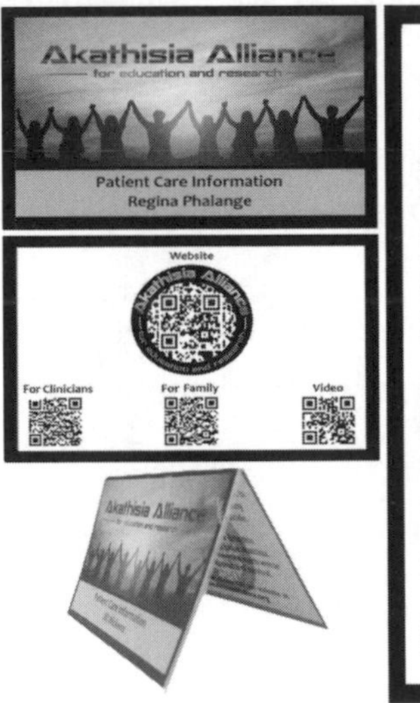

Warning

This patient has a life-threatening condition called akathisia. It is a neurological disorder that causes extreme agitation, inability to remain still, and an overwhelming sense of terror. It is not a mental illness. It is a medication side effect.

Due to the well-documented risk of impulsive suicide, please do not administer dopamine-depleting medications as they can significantly worsen this condition. These include antipsychotics, SSRIs, antiemetics, fluoroquinolone antibiotics, and others.

If this patient is tapering off a benzodiazepine, SSRI, antipsychotic, or another psychotropic medication, it is CRUCIAL to continue their tapering schedule. Any alteration can make their condition much worse.

Most importantly, please do not force medicate this patient with a medication that can cause akathisia or suicidal thoughts as this would significantly increase the likelihood of suicide.

For more information, please visit our website at **https://www.akathisiaalliance.org**

What is Akathisia?

Akathisia is an extremely distressing neurological disorder characterized by severe agitation, an inability to remain still, and an overwhelming sense of terror. These symptoms are so tortuous that it can lead to violence and suicide. Akathisia is primarily caused by prescribed medications. The most frequent offenders are antipsychotics, antidepressants, anti-nausea medications, and antibiotics, but it can be caused by many other medications as well. It is also common in benzodiazepine withdrawal (e.g., Ativan, Klonopin), especially after long-term use. It most often occurs when starting, stopping, or changing the dose of a medication, but it can occur at any time during treatment and even months after it is discontinued. Akathisia is far more common than has been reported in the past and remains dangerously under-diagnosed and under-reported today.

Symptoms

The following common symptoms of akathisia have been reported universally (regardless of whether it was caused by long-term use of a psychiatric medication or by one dose of a non-psychiatric medication):

- Intense physical restlessness with a need for constant movement such as pacing, rocking, foot tapping, hand wringing, and shifting position in a chair
- An overwhelming sense of terror, which has also been described as "chemical terror." This is so pervasive that the person actually feels as if they are experiencing a terrifying event such as being lit on fire or buried alive.
- A feeling often described as wanting to "jump out of my skin"
- Extreme agitation, impatience, and irritability
- Suicidal and/or violent impulses
- Non-suicidal self-harm impulses (e.g., hitting, cutting)
- Depersonalization-derealization (feeling disconnected from the body, as if observing it from the outside, or a sense that the world is unreal, similar to living in a dream)
- Separation anxiety/monophobia and agoraphobia (a need to be near safe people and places at all times due to the terror)
- Racing thoughts and pressured speech
- Vocal tics (e.g., throat clearing, grunting)

- Subjective physical sensations such as electrical zaps, buzzing, vibrating, burning, bugs crawling under the skin, etc.
- Hypersensitivity to light and sound
- Executive dysfunction (impulsivity, disorganization, inattention, emotional dysregulation)

Recognizing Akathisia (ICD-10-CM Code G25.71)

Key Points

- Akathisia is a neurological disorder composed of both neurological and psychological symptoms.
- Motor symptoms can be variable, briefly suppressed, increase with attention, and decrease with distraction.
- Motor symptoms may increase with physical and/or psychological distress.
- Excessive movements are not always evident.
- Due to the above-noted motor characteristics, akathisia can easily be misdiagnosed as a functional neurological disorder.

Clinical Assessment

There is no consensus regarding which movements, if any, are characteristic of akathisia. In our study, the features that best discriminated akathisia from non-akathisia were 1) shifting weight from foot to foot, or walking on the spot, 2) inability to keep legs still (subjectively), 3) feelings of inner restlessness, and 4) shifting of body position in the chair. However, these features are not present in every patient, and in the milder cases, only the subjective report may be present, at least on brief examination, and only prolonged observation will reveal any motor disorder. Voluntary movements and effortful tasks tend to reduce the movements. The majority of the patients report that akathisic movements are voluntary and in response to subjective distress.

Except for the most severe cases, patients are able to voluntarily suppress the movements at least for short periods. Another feature of the movements is their marked variability over time, and their usual disappearance during sleep. Tremor of the extremities is not uncommonly associated, and this may be regarded as the co-occurrence of drug-induced parkinsonism.

Misdiagnosis and Suicidality

Akathisia is not subtle. Its symptoms are so severe, in fact, that there are many reports of people with no history of mental illness or depression who took their lives within days of its onset. The importance of an accurate and swift diagnosis cannot be stressed enough. As the suicidality is primarily due to its subjective symptoms, it is crucial to consider a self-diagnosis—even when a patient exhibits no objective signs. Failure to do so and an alternate misdiagnosis are currently resulting in unnecessary involuntary hospitalizations, forced drugging with medications that worsen the akathisia, loss of family support, abandonment, homelessness, and a much greater risk of suicide.

Common misdiagnoses: Worsening of a mental illness, new mental illness, generalized anxiety disorder, panic disorder, personality disorder, bipolar disorder, attention-deficit/hyperactivity disorder, restless legs syndrome, health anxiety

Functional neurological, somatic symptom, and factitious disorders: Patients with symptoms severe enough to cause suicidality may easily meet the criteria for these disorders until they find a doctor who recognizes their akathisia. They will appear to have disproportionate and persistent thoughts about the seriousness of their symptoms, have a persistently high level of anxiety about their symptoms, and spend excessive time devoted to these symptoms. They will do their own research, know the correct medical terms, be eager to have numerous tests performed, and have a history of visiting many doctors and hospitals.

Drug-seeking: Akathisia is very common in benzodiazepine withdrawal, especially if prescribed long term. It can also occur with tolerance and between doses. To these patients, even one missed dose can cause significant worsening. Due to the increased suicidality, they know they may not survive a cold-turkey withdrawal. They are not drug-seeking to get high. They simply need their prescription renewed so they can taper at a rate slow enough to prevent a return of the akathisia.

Treating Akathisia

Pharmacological treatment of akathisia is extremely difficult because a medication that helps one patient may harm another. Please consult the literature for suggested treatment options. If a patient is tapering off a psychotropic medication, it is crucial to continue their tapering schedule. A faster taper can result in a return, or severe worsening, of their akathisia.

Note: Threatening to restrain and/or force drug patients exhibiting signs of akathisia, including self-harm, could significantly worsen their condition. Using a calm tone to assure them they are safe may be much more effective.

The following dopamine-depleting medications can cause or significantly worsen akathisia:

- aripiprazole (Abilify)
- asenapine (Saphris)
- cariprazine (Vraylar)
- chlorpromazine (Thorazine)
- ciprofloxacin (Cipro)
- citalopram (Celexa)
- clozapine (Clozaril)
- delafloxacin (Baxdela)
- desvenlafaxine (Pristiq)
- domperidone (Motilium)
- doxycycline
- droperidol (Inapsine)
- duloxetine (Cymbalta)
- escitalopram (Lexapro)
- fluoxetine (Prozac)
- fluphenazine (Modecate)
- flupentixol (Fluanxol)
- gemifloxacin (Factive)
- haloperidol (Haldol)
- iloperidone (Fanapt)
- levofloxacin (Levaquin)
- levomilnacipran (Fetzima)
- loxapine (Loxitane)
- lurasidone (Latuda)
- metoclopramide (Reglan)
- milnacipran (Savella)
- moxifloxacin (Avelox)
- ofloxacin (Floxin)
- olanzapine (Zyprexa)
- paliperidone (Invega)
- paroxetine (Paxil)
- perphenazine (Trilafon)
- pimozide (Orap)
- prochlorperazine (Compazine)
- promethazine (Phenergan)
- quetiapine (Seroquel)
- risperidone (Risperdal)
- sertraline (Zoloft)
- thiothixene (Navane)
- tiapride (Tiapridal)
- trifluoperazine (Stelazine)
- trimethobenzamide (Tigan)
- venlafaxine (Effexor)
- ziprasidone (Geodon)
- zuclopenthixol (Clopixol)

Anosognosia or Medication Spellbinding

Personality changes are an adverse effect we might fail to recognize when we are taking antidepressants. This is called "Anosognosia" or "medication spellbinding". The following is how Peter Breggin, psychiatrist and author, describes it, "First, the individuals fail to perceive that they are acting in an irrational, uncharacteristic and dangerous manner. Second, they fail to identify the medication as playing any role in their drastically changed mental processes and activities. Third, they often think that the medication is "helping", although sometimes they believe it's ineffective, and they continue to take it as they deteriorate mentally. In the extreme, individuals suffering from medication-induced mania and psychosis believe that the drug is helping greatly and that they are "better than ever". Fourth, some spellbound individuals become compulsively violent toward themselves or others, and commit bizarre acts wholly alien to their prior personalities."[80]

Coming to terms with our personality, lifestyle or how we behaved whilst taking antidepressants if often one of the most difficult issues to deal with, especially when withdrawing from medication. For some, taking antidepressants has resulted in criminal convictions, relationship breakups, antisocial behavior, financial ruin and what are deemed to be irreparable lives. These are far from uncommon experiences.

Serotonin Syndrome

"Serotonin syndrome" or "serotonin toxicity" is a drug reaction caused by an accumulation of high levels of serotonin. It can be caused by interactions between drugs and by taking too much of the medication or simply when starting, increasing dose or adding a medication. Antidepressants are amongst many drugs and supplements which can cause serotonin syndrome.

We know serotonin influences a wide range of psychological and bodily functions including our central nervous system, brain, blood platelets and intestines and serotonin syndrome is not just about serotonin levels in the brain. It can be mild to life threatening. The main symptoms of serotonin syndrome are agitation or restlessness but can include: confusion, rapid heart rate and high blood pressure, dilated pupils, loss of muscle coordination or twitching muscles, muscle rigidity, heavy sweating, diarrhea, headache, shivering, goose bumps, high fever, seizures, irregular heartbeat and unconsciousness. Severe serotonin syndrome can be life-threatening.

"It's important to stay informed about your medications. Knowing what you are taking, the active ingredients, possible side effects, and medications that should not be mixed are important in avoiding serotonin syndrome. Pay close attention to the instructions of your medications to ensure you are taking them at correct intervals. If you have questions about your medications, reach out to your doctor to double check that you are not mixing medications that could result in serotonin syndrome."[81]

Sex

Sexual problems are one of the most reported adverse effects of antidepressants and are suffered by a significant number of people. They can cause a wide range of symptoms including, erectile dysfunction, inability to orgasm, pleasureless orgasm, diminished libido, genital numbness.

"They should be called anti-sex drugs rather than antidepressant drugs," says Jon Jureidini, a child psychiatrist of 30 years standing, a professor of psychiatry and pediatrics at the University of Adelaide and co-author of a BMJ study, "It's more reliably predictable that they're going to get rid of sexual function than it is that they're going to get rid of depression." Some people find this persists long after they cease taking the drug. "Post-SSRI sexual dysfunction (PSSD) is an iatrogenic condition which can arise following antidepressant use, in which sexual function does not completely return to normal after the discontinuation of SSRIs, SNRIs and some tricyclic antidepressants."[82]

Manufacturer information about this is sometimes buried, or misleading. It is believed that many people who take antidepressants for a significant length of time will be guaranteed to experience sexual adverse effects. If we realized this, we might not be so quick to fill our prescription, especially at a young age.

Sexual problems are one of the most common reasons people would like to stop their medication and this should always be done with a competent medical professional or support service. Online advice, such as the following often suggests we can "take a drug holiday" but this should definitely be avoided.

"Taking a drug holiday. Depending on how long the drug usually remains in your body, you might stop taking it for a few days—for example, before a weekend, if that's when you hope to have sex. This isn't spontaneous, but it can work if you carefully follow your doctor's directions about how to stop and resume your medication. However, there is always a chance that this might cause a relapse, especially if it is one of the drugs that leaves your system relatively rapidly."[83]

This is incredibly bad advice and taking a drug holiday should never be an option. Stopping abruptly at any time can be dangerous, even if it is "for a few days"! Rather than causing a "relapse", our sex-induced antidepressant break could cause life threatening withdrawal symptoms.

Alcohol

The relationship between alcohol and antidepressants is unknown. However, we are generally advised not to drink alcohol with antidepressants as alcohol can make depression worse, increase anxiety, and cause personality changes. It is thought mixing antidepressants and alcohol can also lead to worse adverse effects of the medication. Some report alcohol can even prevent antidepressants working properly. What we do know is many people who take antidepressants become alcohol dependent or abuse alcohol. A combination of antidepressants and alcohol can be devastating. Anecdotal evidence tells us alcohol problems often begin soon after a person starts to take antidepressants.

The 2014 study "Ninety-three cases of alcohol dependence following SSRI treatment" looked at reports linking serotonin reuptake inhibitor use with increased alcohol consumption.

It concluded, "The data make it clear that all treatments with significant effects on the serotonin reuptake system are likely to cause this problem. Both sexes, and all ages are affected, and reports have come from a range of countries. SSRI induced alcoholism is likely to be a relatively common problem. Recognizing the problem can lead to a gratifying cure. A failure to recognize it can be fatal."[84]

Reports link antidepressants and cravings for alcohol, in particular paroxetine.[85] Experienced with anosognosia, the effects of alcohol can have devastating effects on our lives. Many of us do not realize antidepressants are causing our problems with alcohol and the combination can cause life changing uncharacteristic behavior.

Pregnancy

It has been referred to as a "pre-pregnancy dilemma" but it is not as simple as do we stay on antidepressants or stop taking them. If we want to have a baby.[86] Without realizing it many young women will have already become dependent on their antidepressants and may not be able to stop them if they want to. Those who try due to pregnancy, often do so unsupervised and without tapering slowly and find themselves with horrendous withdrawal symptoms. The doctor will say this is a "relapse" and prescribe more antidepressants! If they try to taper during pregnancy, lasting withdrawal effects might be confused with postpartum depression. A dilemma indeed!

Women in the US are twice as likely as men to take antidepressants. "During 2008–2013, approximately 15% of a convenience sample of reproductive-aged women (aged 15–44 years) with employer-sponsored insurance filled a prescription for antidepressants. The most commonly filled antidepressants were sertraline, bupropion, and citalopram."[87]

Taking antidepressants whilst pregnant is a worrying issue for many. We will probably be told the risks of not treating depression outweigh the risks of antidepressants to both mother and baby, but we do know antidepressants can cross the placenta and enter the amniotic fluid. They can also be found in breastmilk. There is an increasing amount of compelling evidence that an antidepressant free pregnancy might be our best option.

Studies show one in every three babies born to mothers on antidepressants will have mild symptoms which can include jitteriness, poor feeding, agitation and fast breathing. There is also a slightly increased risk of Persistent Pulmonary Hypertension (PPHN) in the newborn. PPHN is a very rare but potentially very serious problem causing breathing difficulties.[88]

A 2014 study in Canada, looked at infants born over a decade. It found a link between women taking SSRI drugs and an increased risk of autism in their children. "Use of antidepressants, specifically SSRIs, during the second and/or third trimester increases the risk of autism spectrum disorder in children, even after considering maternal depression."[89]

A US study reported some birth defects occur 2–3.5 times more frequently among the infants of women who took paroxetine or fluoxetine early in pregnancy. The CDC study findings refute some of the earlier reported links but confirm other links observed between birth defects and some SSRI antidepressants.

Researchers still observed five out of the seven previous links between paroxetine and certain birth defects. In the study, paroxetine appeared to be linked with these birth defects:

- Anencephaly, a birth defect of a baby's brain and skull
- Atrial septal defects, a type of heart defect
- Heart defects with obstruction of the right ventricular outflow tract
- Gastroschisis, a birth defect of the abdominal wall
- Omphalocele, another type of birth defect of the abdominal wall

Despite the increased risks for certain birth defects from some SSRIs found in this study, the actual risk for a birth defect among babies born to women taking one of these medications is still very low.[90]

We should never stop taking antidepressants suddenly, even if we discover we are pregnant. It is important we consult our doctor and discuss our options. It is however, one issue which young women need to think about when they consider taking antidepressants, even if pregnancy might not be at the forefront of their minds.

Drug Interactions

"It is important to be aware of common drug interactions between SSRIs and other medications, especially because some SSRIs are competitive inhibitors of a variety of cytochrome P450 liver enzymes. Therefore, they can significantly increase the blood levels of medications that are metabolized by those liver enzymes. Drug interactions with clinical consequences usually involve combinations of an SSRI with other psychotropics, especially monoamine oxidase inhibitors (MAOIs) and tricyclic antidepressants. The interaction between MAOIs and SSRIs is the most important drug interaction limiting SSRI use. MAOI's are infrequently prescribed due to other options available and the high risk of interaction with other drugs."[91]

To avoid serotonin syndrome antidepressants should not be taken with other drugs which increase serotonin activity. There are certain other drugs SSRIs should not be mixed with. Amongst these are the herbal St. John's wort, monoamine oxidase inhibitors such as phenelzine (Nardil), and clomipramine (Anafranil), tramadol and meperidine. Serotonin syndrome has also been reported when an SSRI is combined with lithium. Sertraline, citalopram and escitalopram have the lowest potential for drug interactions.

Drug Interaction Checker

The RxISK website has a drug interaction checker we can use to check if our antidepressants might interact with other medication.

This tool, available at rxisk.org/tools/drug-interaction-checker, uses the following resources provided by the US National Library of Medicine:

- ONCHigh is a list of high-priority drug-drug interactions derived by a panel of experts and contained in a JAMIA article.
- DrugBank contains the drug-drug interactions contained in the DrugBank database.

This interaction checker is not intended as a substitute for professional medical advice, diagnosis, or treatment.[92]

10
ANTIDEPRESSANT-INDUCED SUICIDE

Can antidepressants make us suicidal and why do suicide prevention experts choose to ignore prescription drug-induced suicide?

A paradoxical reaction or paradoxical effect is an effect of medical treatment, usually a drug, opposite to the effect which would normally be expected. An example of a paradoxical reaction is suicidal ideation caused by antidepressants. It is now widely acknowledged that prescription drugs can put us at risk of dangerous adverse effects, most notably that antidepressants and some other medication can raise the risk of suicide.

Animal studies demonstrate, when initially given fluoxetine the brain actually shuts down its own production of serotonin, causing a paradoxical effect or opposite effect on the level of serotonin.[93] The brain's chemistry wants to remain balanced and any disruption from SSRIs or other medications throws the brain off balance. What results from this disturbance is often described as being like a "rollercoaster effect". A person's mood can go from consistently depressed to temporarily content, to all over the place very quickly. This is why "Black Box Warnings" are required on all SSRIs.[94]

Suicide risk with antidepressants has previously been falsely reported in pharmaceutical industry trials but recent research published in the Journal of Psychotherapy and Psychosomatics reports adults prescribed antidepressants for depression are 2.5 times more likely to attempt suicide when compared to those taking a placebo. Conducted by

Dr. Michael P. Hengartner, a senior research fellow at the Zurich University of Applied Sciences and Dr. Martin Plöderl, a senior researcher at Paracelsus Medical University, Salzburg, the study, "Newer-generation antidepressants and suicide risk in randomized controlled trials: A re-analysis of the FDA database" found 1 in every 200 people who start treatment will attempt suicide due to the effects of the drug.[95] They examined all suicides and suicide attempts recorded in the safety summaries of all antidepressant trials submitted to the US drug regulator FDA, between 1987 and 2013, for marketing authorization of new antidepressant drugs for the treatment of adult major depression. In these randomized controlled clinical trials, the rate of suicide was about three times higher in those taking antidepressants compared to a placebo, and the rate of non-fatal suicide attempts and suicides combined was about 2.5 times higher in those taking antidepressants compared to placebo.

Akathisia, the drug-induced state of acute physical and psychological agitation, puts patients at risk of suicide in two ways. Rather than contemplating and planning suicide, akathisia often presents people with a tortuous fight to stay alive. This severe anxiety, restlessness, agitation, psychosis-like state can mean we have little control over our mind and suicidal impulses and thoughts are outside our control. In other cases, it can be so uncomfortable and so distressing, accompanied by other severe physical adverse effects that people often turn to suicide as their only option.

Many akathisia sufferers have called charities and suicide lines only to be misunderstood and asked, "What is wrong with you?" These are often people in the high-risk groups; young and middle-aged men, people in the care of mental health services, people in the criminal justice system, doctors, nurses, veterans and people with a history of antidepressant induced self-harm. Nearly always they are people who are starting, changing dose or withdrawing from psychotropic medication. They are people suffering from prescription drug reactions and find no help from the medical profession or from charity help lines.

Admittedly most doctors and healthcare workers do not understand akathisia and the symptoms of anxiety, agitation or suicidality are often diagnosed as a recurrence or worsening of illness, rather than a drug-induced adverse event. Suicide-inducing akathisia, an adverse reaction to antidepressants and other psychiatric drugs is overlooked in medical error, willfully ignored by governments and suicide prevention organizations, and all the while it is an avoidable adverse reaction of prescribed medication. (Psychiatric drugs are not the only drugs that cause akathisia. People who take drugs such as anti-emetics (anti-nausea drugs), antibiotics, antipsychotics and opioids, may also experience akathisia and become suicidal—people who do not in any way have identifiable psychiatric disorders).[96]

Peter Breggin, leading psychiatrist and medical expert who has examined dozens of cases of individuals who have died by suicide or committed violent crimes whilst under the influence of SSRIs says, "certain behaviors are known to be associated with these drugs, including anxiety, agitation, panic attacks, insomnia, irritability, hostility, impulsivity, akathisia (severe restlessness), hypomania, and mania. Any of these adverse effects, including emotional blunting, can cause both suicide and violence.[97]

In the US, the national rate of suicide has risen 33% over the past two decades. A 2016 study reported suicides and suicide attempts cost $93.5 billion a year, most of it in lost productivity.[98] Decades of research into suicide prevention has been done and there are still no effective prevention strategies. Little scientific evidence exists that media campaigns and government strategies reduce suicide and mounting evidence that they don't.

Mental health conditions are said to be "one of several contributors to suicide." So why are antidepressants and their paradoxical effects hardly ever mentioned? If governments, charities and suicide prevention organizations really want to address the issue of suicide, why do they fail to mention prescription medication as a leading cause and overlook the opportunity to reduce suicide caused by medicalization? Despite Black Box Warnings, why does prescription medication, in particular psychiatric drugs, remain a taboo subject for suicide prevention experts?

Researchers reported on a study of suicide rates in 76 countries. They found suicides were higher in countries with mental health legislation. They reported there was a correlation between higher suicide rates and a higher number of psychiatric beds, psychiatrists and psychiatric nurses, more mental health training for primary care professionals and greater spending on mental health as a percentage of total spending on health in the country. It all points to the medicalization of suicide.[101]

In 2020, September 10 was designated Suicide Prevention Day and was piously promoted as an exercise in increased awareness. Yet if it really were a "piously promoted" Suicide Prevention Day, there would have been mention in the media of one of the main causes of suicide: psychiatric medications including SSRI/SNRI antidepressants. These medications have destroyed many lives. It is well established that they cause suicidality in some people—people who are not depressed—yet in all the media hoopla about suicide prevention, these medications taken by millions, are seemingly irrelevant.

SSRI Stories is a website with over 7,000 stories mentioning antidepressants. Most of them have been published in newspapers or scientific journals. It seems clear that antidepressants contributed to the tragic outcomes of the individuals involved. The stories include violence, suicide, serious adverse reactions, personality changes, etc.

"The media used to know how damaging these medications can be. Stories from the 1990s on this website prove that. But after years of marketing of psych meds, and years of lawsuits failing because of system flaws, the media now go along with the pharma mantra that antidepressants save lives. There is not a shred of evidence that this is true, and plenty of evidence that these drugs cause enormous harm. But the press that supposedly prides itself in unbiased reporting simply chooses not to know."[102]

Rather than being presented with the following article in the New York Times, "Is the Pandemic Sparking Suicide? Psychiatrists are confronted with an urgent natural experiment, and the outcome is far from predictable",[103] shouldn't we be asking "With the alarming increase in psychiatric drug prescribing, are we confronted with an urgent natural experiment or a medical trend we are purposely choosing to ignore?"

FDA Medication Guide: Antidepressants and Suicide

Medication Guide Antidepressant Medicines, Depression and other Serious Mental Illnesses, and Suicidal Thoughts or Actions

Read the Medication Guide that comes with you or your family member's antidepressant medicine. This Medication Guide is only about the risk of suicidal thoughts and actions with antidepressant medicines.

Talk to your (or your family member's) healthcare provider about:

- all risks and benefits of treatment with antidepressant medicines
- all treatment choices for depression or other serious mental illness

What is the most important information I should know about antidepressant medicines, depression and other serious mental illnesses, and suicidal thoughts or actions?

1. Antidepressant medicines may increase suicidal thoughts or actions in some children, teenagers, and young adults within the first few months of treatment.
2. Depression and other serious mental illnesses are the most important causes of suicidal thoughts and actions. Some people may have a particularly high risk of having suicidal thoughts or actions. These include people who have (or have a family history of) bipolar illness (also called manic depressive illness) or suicidal thoughts or actions.
3. How can I watch for and try to prevent suicidal thoughts and actions in myself or a family member?
    a. Pay close attention to any changes, especially sudden changes, in mood, behaviors, thoughts, or feelings. This is very important when an antidepressant medicine is started or when the dose is changed.
    b. Call the healthcare provider right away to report new or sudden changes in mood, behavior, thoughts, or feelings.
    c. Keep all follow-up visits with the healthcare provider as scheduled. Call the healthcare provider between visits as needed, especially if you have concerns about symptoms.

Call a healthcare provider right away if you or your family member has any of the following symptoms, especially if they are new, worse, or worry you:

- thoughts about suicide or dying
- acting on dangerous impulses
- attempts to commit suicide

- an extreme increase in activity and new or worse depression talking (mania)
- new or worse anxiety
- other unusual changes in behavior or feeling very agitated or restless mood
- panic attacks
- trouble sleeping (insomnia)
- new or worse irritability
- acting aggressive, being angry, or violent

What else do I need to know about antidepressant medicines?

- Never stop an antidepressant medicine without first talking to a healthcare provider. Stopping an antidepressant medicine suddenly can cause other symptoms.
- Antidepressants are medicines used to treat depression and other illnesses. It is important to discuss all the risks of treating depression and also the risks of not treating it. Patients and their families or other caregivers should discuss all treatment choices with the healthcare provider, not just the use of antidepressants.
- Antidepressant medicines have other side effects. Talk to the healthcare provider about the side effects of the medicine prescribed for you or your family member.
- Antidepressant medicines can interact with other medicines. Know all of the medicines that you or your family member takes. Keep a list of all medicines to show the healthcare provider. Do not start new medicines without first checking with your healthcare provider.
- Not all antidepressant medicines prescribed for children are FDA approved for use in children. Talk to your child's healthcare provider for more information. This Medication Guide has been approved by the U.S. Food and Drug Administration for all antidepressants.[104]

First an antidepressant, then the "side" effects and then one drug leads to another and another... and another...

> *"The last thing you want to do is use one drug to treat the adverse effects of another... initially it might seem to work but just like any other prescribed medication that causes dependence over time it will make things exponentially worse."*

In the New York Times article, "The Risks of the Prescribing Cascade,"[105] Jane E. Brody explains, "The problem occurs when drug-induced side effects are viewed as a new ailment and treated with yet another drug that can cause still other side effects." She describes the case of the 87-year old mother of a pharmacist who was repeatedly misdiagnosed and inappropriately prescribed medications.

Antidepressants are often gateway drugs to polypharmacy (being prescribed and taking multiple medications), what Brody describes as "a costly and often frightening medically induced condition called "a prescribing cascade" that starts with drug-induced side effects which are then viewed as a new ailment and treated with yet another drug or drugs that can cause still other side effects." With antidepressants it can mean multiple psychiatric drugs, or any other classes of drug are prescribed, often off-label, to treat any of the hundreds of adverse effects listed in the Patient Information Leaflets.

If we consider the number of possible adverse effects antidepressants can have, it is easy to see why their risks might be greater than their benefits. Antidepressants affect different people in different ways, and it is very common for us to become a victim of polypharmacy if the adverse effects go unrecognized or misdiagnosed as a new condition. The potential to be prescribed more medication is an important reason why we need to be savvy and aware of the adverse effects of antidepressants. Recognizing, making our prescriber aware of, and questioning our adverse effects can prevent further conditions being diagnosed and more unnecessary medication added to our drug regimen.

Thankfully, questions are starting to be asked about prescribers' knowledge of drug adverse effects and how we, the patients can educate ourselves. "So I started to wonder: How much knowledge do doctors have about medications? What can patients do to educate and protect themselves?"[106] It is now recognized doctors might be underreporting to the FDA's voluntary Adverse Event Reporting System.

A welcome development is PIMsPlus which has been developed with the Department of Family Medicine at McMaster University, the American Society of Consultant Pharmacists, and TaperMD, "to address the serious problems of polypharmacy, prescribing cascades, and drug side effects. All of the collaborators contribute to the development and maintenance of PIMsPLUS at their own expense."[107]

It is crucial we avoid unnecessary medication but unless we become our own experts, we are vulnerable to becoming a multi-medicated, revolving door patient with pills for every adverse effect and adverse effects for every pill.

11
ANTIDEPRESSANTS AND OUR "MEDICALLY UNEXPLAINED SYMPTOMS"

What happens when our adverse effects are labelled "Medically Unexplained Symptoms"? Why do so many doctors fail to recognize antidepressants are causing our symptoms and diagnose additional conditions and illnesses?

Treatment from our doctors for our mental health is most likely to be a prescription for antidepressants, which most believe to be safe and effective, or, at worst, no better than placebo. However, antidepressants result in homeostatic effects which medically adjust our serotonin system. These drugs cross the blood-brain barrier and have all sorts of unintended consequences. "Most serotonin is found outside the central nervous system, and virtually all of the 15 serotonin receptors are expressed outside as well as within the brain. Serotonin regulates numerous biological processes including cardiovascular function, bowel motility, ejaculatory latency, and bladder control."[108,109]

Rather than simply correcting a serotonin imbalance in our brain, taking antidepressants creates all sorts of knock-on effects as they mess with serotonin. These are described by Kelly Brogan in her article, "What's the harm in taking an antidepressant?" in which she summarizes the ground-breaking 2016 research, "The Safety, Tolerability and Risks Associated with the Use of Newer Generation Antidepressant Drugs."[110]

Some people are unable to metabolize antidepressants and may develop adverse reactions which can be serious. These should, hopefully, be recognized quickly and the drug very gradually reduced and stopped before more harm is done. As we know, most people will be encouraged to struggle through the first few weeks of treatment until they "adjust to" the drug. Many of us can feel emotionally numbed by the drugs—but also develop physical symptoms such as sexual dysfunction, gut issues, weight gain, fatigue etc., which can be explained as side effects of the drugs being taken as prescribed. Unfortunately, many doctors fail to recognize our genuine physical or psychological symptoms as the adverse effects of antidepressants and they might tell us we are wrong to put our symptoms down to the antidepressants we are taking. Others will look for alternative explanations resulting in a series of examinations and investigations which will generally produce negative results.

If we see our doctor because of what we believe might be the adverse effects of antidepressants, it is very common for doctors to tell us we are suffering "medically unexplained", somatic or functional symptoms (MUS). These symptoms, which doctors might describe as "of unknown etiology" (meaning the cause is unknown), often lead to a diagnosis such as Chronic Fatigue Syndrome (CFS), Irritable Bowel Syndrome (IBS), Fibromyalgia or Myalgic Encephalomyelitis (ME). As with our first "mental illness" diagnosis, there are rarely any investigative tools or tests that can confirm the presence of these new illnesses. Medically Unexplained Symptoms is, however, becoming a growing field of research and development as professionals capitalize on the opportunities the adverse effects of antidepressants present.

Doctors have been trained to prescribe antidepressants using the PHQ-9 and GAD-7 questionnaires and during antidepressant treatment they might also use the PHQ-15 questionnaire to "diagnose" any subsequent developments of new symptoms and suffering as "psychosomatic".

Antidepressant withdrawal/discontinuation symptoms were recognized in the 1990s by researchers using the DESS (Discontinuation-Emergent Signs and Symptoms scale). In the early 2000s this list of very debilitating symptoms was divided up and re-branded (with funding from Pfizer).[111]

Doctors, psychiatrists, psychologists and therapists frequently believe patients are "somatising"; (experiencing psychological distress in the form of physical symptoms), when many of us are actually suffering the serious physical effects of commonly prescribed and supposedly safe and effective antidepressants. These effects are dangerously unrecognized or ignored by prescribers, sometimes with serious consequences. Doctors can become frustrated when we keep going to see them with "functional", "somatic" or "Medically Unexplained Symptoms" (MUS). Medically Unexplained Symptoms are becoming a growing burden on and are stretching health service resources.[112]

PHYSICAL SYMPTOMS (PHQ-15)			
During the past 4 weeks, how much have you been bothered by any of the following problems?	**Not bothered at all**	**Bothered a little**	**Bothered a lot**
a. Stomach pain	0	1	2
b. Back pain	0	1	2
c. Pain in your arms, legs, or joints (knees, hips, etc.)	0	1	2
d. Menstrual cramps or other problems with your periods (WOMEN ONLY)	0	1	2
e. Headaches	0	1	2
f. Chest pain	0	1	2
g. Dizziness	0	1	2
h. Fainting spells	0	1	2
i. Feeling your heart pound or race	0	1	2
j. Shortness of breath	0	1	2
k. Pain or problems during sexual intercourse	0	1	2
l. Constipation, loose bowels, or diarrhea	0	1	2
m. Nausea, gas, or indigestion	0	1	2
n. Feeling tired or having low energy	0	1	2
o. Trouble sleeping	0	1	2
	add columns:	______	+ ______

(For office coding): TOTAL SCORE = ☐

Developed by Drs. Robert L. Spitzer, Janet B.W. Williams, Kurt Kroenke and colleagues, with an educational grant from Pfizer Inc. No permission required to reproduce, translate, display or distribute.

In 2013, the American Psychiatric Association rejected the term "Medically Unexplained Symptoms" in its Diagnostic and Statistical Manual (DSM-5), replacing it with "somatization" and "somatic symptom disorder". This refers to excessive thoughts, feelings, or behaviors related to somatic (physical) symptoms or health concerns. "We tried to get away from saying whether the symptoms are explained or not, and just allow people to have symptoms," said Michael Sharpe, MD, a University of Oxford psychiatrist who studies the psychological aspects of medical illness. Dr. Sharpe was on the DSM-5 work group for somatic symptoms. So, it seems they decided to "just allow patients to have symptoms" with no reference to the possibility the symptoms might be the adverse effects of medication. When our symptoms become severe or chronic, they then become a "disorder".[113] The category "somatic symptom disorder" is for people with severe, chronic and troublesome physical symptoms that may or may not have a medical explanation. Medically unexplained symptoms can be classified as a psychiatric disorder and patients' symptoms are attributed to their underlying anxiety or depression—or whatever they may or may not have been suffering when started on antidepressants. Doctors are failing to recognize that these multiple serious physical symptoms are actually due to taking or withdrawing from antidepressants—and this obscures, covers up and misinterprets what is really happening to people.

It is about so much more than "just allowing us to have symptoms", it is about ignoring the adverse effects of medication and opportunistically classifying them as illnesses. It is, in some ways, a very similar process to mental health "illncss" diagnosis. In the British Medical Journal (BMJ), Allen Frances warned "the DSM-5 introduces a poorly tested diagnosis—somatic symptom disorder—which risks mislabeling a sizeable proportion of the population as mentally ill."[114] Marion Brown, Psychotherapist, responded in the BMJ, "Something is going horribly wrong when it is becoming apparent that previously healthy patients are being seriously harmed and made very unwell by medicines 'taken as prescribed' -and are then being dismissed/described as troublesome heartsink patients who display 'excessive' responses to distressing, chronic, somatic symptoms with associated dysfunctional thoughts, feelings, or behaviors. These patients are finding their medical records and referral letters -and even reports to

MHRA -couched in phrases such as 'the patient believes,' and 'the patient thinks.' They are also being labelled with 'attention seeking behaviors' and assorted 'personality disorders' so as to discount and deny credibility of their very real experiences and immensely distressing functional symptoms."[115]

It is estimated about 1 in 4 people who see their GP in the UK have Medically Unexplained Symptoms and 1 in 3 patients or more in a neurological outpatient setting. The UK Royal College of Psychiatrists say, "Other diagnoses can be given for medically unexplained symptoms, but it is common to use a general term to describe the symptoms, such as "medically unexplained symptoms." Another common term is "functional;" i.e., the symptoms are due to a problem in the way the body is functioning, even though the structure of the body is norm." Amongst their treatment recommendations are antidepressants, the very source of many medically unexplained symptoms; "Antidepressants are used to treat a range of problems, not just depression, and can help treat medically unexplained symptoms in a number of ways."[116] The Royal College of Psychiatrists do not wish to acknowledge "the problem in the way the body is functioning" might very well be due to the effects of antidepressants or other medication the patient might be taking. Their solution is to recommend prescribing more antidepressants as the answer to relieving the medically unexplained symptoms they have potentially caused!

If we look at the Patient Information Leaflet for SSRI and SNRI antidepressants, we will find every symptom listed on the PHQ-15 is also listed as a possible side effect of antidepressants! Stomach problems, nausea, joint pain, menstrual problems, headaches, chest pain, dizziness and fainting, heart palpitations, shortness of breath sexual problems, tiredness and trouble sleeping are ALL listed as possible side effects of antidepressants in the Patient Information Leaflets.[117]

A more realistic representation of Medically Unexplained Symptoms is shown in Marion Brown's "A Patient's journey. Consequences of Antidepressants/Benzodiazepines".[118]

If anything demonstrates "a wicked problem whose social complexity means that it has no determinable stopping point" and "because of complex interdependencies the effort to solve one aspect of the 'wicked' problem may reveal or create other problems", then the industry created concept of "medically unexplained symptoms" is it![119]

A PATIENT'S JOURNEY

Consequences of Antidepressants/Benzodiazepines

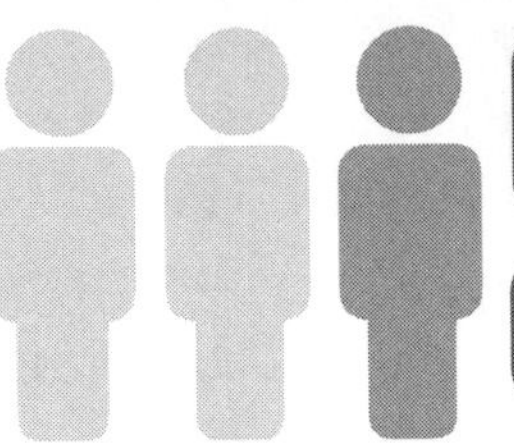

LIFE CRISIS AND/OR TRAUMA FEELING OVERWHELMED

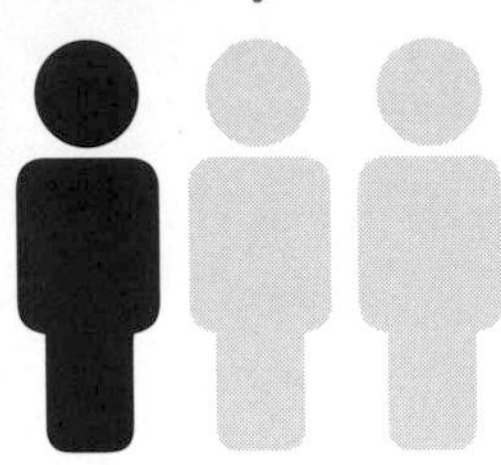

Insomnia, anxiety, panic, anger, depressed, not coping

VISIT EFFECTIVE THERAPIST

TELL STORY - FEEL HEARD & VALIDATED

Psychoeducation, understanding

Breathing, Guided Imagery

Trauma recognised/healing

PATIENT RETURNS TO LIFE - NEEDS MET

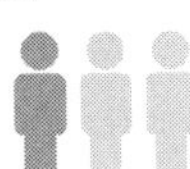

VISIT GP

Started on antidepressants (AD) or benzodiazepines (BZ)

GP advises: Stay on ADs for **AT LEAST SIX MONTHS**

Patient wishes to stop

GP advises rapid taper

Withdrawal symptoms

Doctor misdiagnoses relapse, puts patient back on ADs/BZs

No response or adverse effects = dosage increased or other drugs added

Patient unable to stop, seeks help elsewhere

SLOW TAPER

Patient may or may not get off the drugs

Withdrawal problems

Protracted syndrome

Multiple physical symptoms

Patient seeks medical advice

GP blames underlying condition

Patient undergoes extensive and costly tests

GP/Specialist diagnoses Medically Unexplained Symptoms (MUS)

Functional Somatic Syndromes

Treated with CBT/Graded exercise

Potentially given ADs

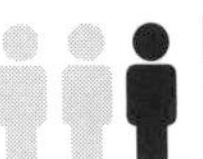

Patient disabled with no understanding and little support

Concept: Marion Brown, 2018. Design by: Miranda, **miranda-design.co.uk**

A PATIENT'S JOURNEY

Consequences of Antidepressants/Benzodiazepines

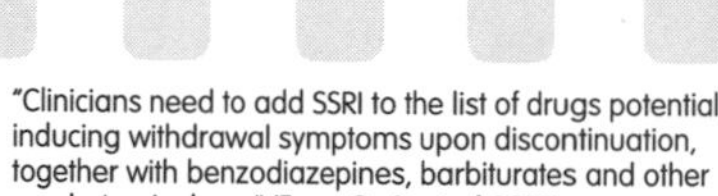

"Clinicians need to add SSRI to the list of drugs potentially inducing withdrawal symptoms upon discontinuation, together with benzodiazepines, barbiturates and other psychotropic drugs" **(Fava G. A. et al 2015)**

SIGNS AND SYMPTOMS OF WITHDRAWAL FROM SSRI
(www.karger.com/Article/FullText/370338)

SYSTEM INVOLVED	SYMPTOMS
General	Flu-like symptoms, fatigue, weakness, tiredness, headache, tachycardia, dyspnea
Balance	Gait instability, ataxia, dizziness, light headedness, vertigo
Sensory	Paraesthesias, electric-shock sensations, myalgias, neuralgias, tinnitus, altered taste, pruritus
Visual	Visual changes, blurred vision
Neuromotor	Tremor, myoclonus, ataxia, muscle rigidity, jerkiness, muscle aches, facial numbness
Vasomotor	Sweating, flushing, chills
Sleep	Insomnia, vivid dreams, nightmares, hypersomnia, lethargy
Gastrointestinal	Nausea, vomiting, diarrhea, anorexia, abdominal pain
Affective	Anxiety, agitation, tension, panic, depression, intensification of suicidal ideation, irritability, impulsiveness, aggression, anger, bouts of crying, mood swings, derealization and depersonalization
Psychotic	Visual and auditory hallucinations
Cognitive	Confusion, decreased concentration, amnesia
Sexual	Genital hypersensitivity, premature ejaculation

What is MUS?

"Medically Unexplained Symptoms (MUS) refers to persistent bodily complaints for which adequate examination does not reveal sufficiently explanatory structural or other specified pathology. MUS are common, with a spectrum of severity, and patients are found in all areas of the healthcare system.

Patients with MUS are more likely to attribute their illness to physical causes rather than lifestyle factors. This can include symptoms such as pain in different parts of the body, functional disturbance of organ systems and complaints of fatigue or exhaustion."

FUNCTIONAL SOMATIC SYNDROMES

SYMPTOMS (COMBINATION OF)	SYNDROME
Bloating, constipation, loose stools, abdominal pain	Irritable Bowel Syndrome
Fatigue (particularly post-exertional and long recovery) pain, sensitivity to smell	Chronic Fatigue Syndrome, Myalgic Encephalomyelitis
Headache, vomiting, dizziness	Post Concussion Syndrome
Pelvic pain, painful sex, painful periods	Chronic pelvic pain
Pain and tender joints, fatigue	Fibromyalgia/Chronic widespread pain
Chest pain, palpitations, shortness of breath	Non cardiac chest pain
Shortness of breath	Hyperventilation
Jaw pain, teeth grinding	Temporo-mandibular Joint Dysfunction
Reaction to smells, light	Multiple Chemical Sensitivity

Source: Joint Commissioning Panel for mental health, Guidance MUS, Feb 2017, www.jcpmh.info

NOTE THE CLEAR SIMILARITIES IN THE SYMPTOMS OF WITHDRAWAL AND 'UNEXPLAINED' SYMPTOMS

Concept: Marion Brown, 2018. Design by: Miranda, **miranda-design.co.uk**

12
BECOMING OUR OWN ANTIDEPRESSANT EXPERT

We need to adopt an approach where one of the first questions we ask is: "Could it be my medication?" This approach should also be adopted by everyone who has a responsibility for our health care.

> *"Patients need to become their own experts, researching drugs on websites—such as the government database MedlinePlus—that are 'free of [the pharmaceutical] industry. Doctors have a responsibility to listen to their patients about side effects, too, she said. I tell medical students: If a patient develops a symptom after they've gone on their drug, it's always the drug's fault until proven otherwise. We're in sort of a bad situation now where the people in control of prescribing drugs know the least about the drugs."*[120]

In an ideal world, when it comes to our health care, we should all try to become our own experts. In the real world, not everyone is in a position where we can. Learning as much as we can about our medication and the possible adverse effects is a start. There are many ways we can do this including books, websites and video links listed in the resource section of this book.

The FDA advises, "Be an active member of your health care team. By taking time to learn about the possible side effects of a drug and working with your health care provider and pharmacist, you will be better prepared to reduce your chance of experiencing a side effect or coping with any side effect that you may experience."[121] They encourage side effects to be reported to FDA's MedWatch, a program for reporting serious problems with human medical products.[122]

Back in the real world of adverse effects, the most useful website is RxISK. Their mission is "Making medicines safer for all of us."[123] It is owned by Data Based Medicine Americas Ltd. (DBM), based in Toronto and run by internationally renowned medical experts including Dr. David Healy, Dr. Dee Mangin, and Dr. Kalman Applbaum.[124] RxISK's goals are educating and empowering patients to have better conversations about their medications with their doctors and collecting data on the unintended consequences of prescription medications so that they can draw attention to them. The website includes a "Drug search" where we can find out about the adverse effects of our medication. It includes MedlinePlus Consumer Information (U.S. NLM).[125]

13
ANTIDEPRESSANT LONG-TERM EFFECTS

Little research exists on the outcomes of people taking antidepressants long-term. Might we suffer significantly worse outcomes if we choose to stay on them?

The National Institute of Mental Health (NIMH), say people regularly recover from depression without having a second episode, for example Jonathan Cole in 1964, "Depression is, on the whole, one of the psychiatric conditions with the best prognosis for eventual recovery, with or without treatment." Given this understanding of the natural course of depression, the NIMH's experts believed that antidepressants might shorten the time to recovery, but they wouldn't be able to boost long-term recovery rates. In 1974, Dean Schuyler, head of the depression section at the NIMH, explained that most depressive episodes "will run their course and terminate with virtually complete recovery without specific intervention."[127] Michael Posternak, psychiatrist at Brown University wrote, "If as many as 85% of depressed individuals who go without somatic treatment spontaneously recover within one year, it would be extremely difficult for any intervention to demonstrate a superior result to this."[128]

"What are the long-term implications of taking antidepressants? The truth of the matter is that it's hard to really know because we don't do placebo-controlled trials for 20 years. We treat people and if they're in a controlled trial, it lasts 12 weeks, maybe 6 months if you stretch it. How do you sort out the effects of the medication from the effects of the disease or from the effects of a lot of other things? These are hard questions to answer." Dr. John Campo, chair of the department of Psychiatry and Behavioral Health at The Ohio State University Wexner Medical Center.[129]

Doctors rarely warn us about the long-term effects of antidepressant use and it is something most of us fail to consider when first starting treatment. There are many of us who have continued to take antidepressants since the early 1990s and the emergence of SSRIs and the chemical imbalance theory. There are now many concerns regarding long-term antidepressant use and the lack of research. The few available studies suggest all the major antidepressants add little additional long-term benefit, and for some patients they may lead to significantly worse long-term outcomes. It is now feared that long-term antidepressant users might be risking permanent damage to our brains and general health.[130]

This is definitely one of the reasons, if we choose to take antidepressants, we should limit the time we take them to the shortest possible. As people stay on antidepressants longer, we are seeing some of the effects of the drugs could be permanent. There are emerging concerns regarding long-term antidepressant use and it is really only from anecdotal evidence that we are starting to learn some of these effects. We desperately need ongoing evaluation of antidepressant benefits and their potential long-term risk of causing certain illnesses. One thing seems certain, antidepressants and other psychotropic drugs do not reduce the number of chronically ill patients in society. If antidepressants cure depression, why do so many of us remain depressed and why do so many who take them have a poor quality of life?

US science journalist Robert Whitaker tells us, in "Anatomy of an Epidemic", the increasing use of drugs not only keeps patients stuck in the sick role, but also turns many problems that would have been transient into chronic diseases.[131] In Psychology Today, he describes Giovanna Fava's 1994 recently reviewed research, "Can long-term treatment with antidepressant drugs worsen the course of depression?" Fava concludes, "There is increasing awareness that, in some cases, long-term use of antidepressant drugs (AD) may enhance the biochemical vulnerability to depression and worsen its long-term outcome and symptomatic expression, decreasing both the likelihood of subsequent response to pharmacological treatment and the duration of symptom-free periods."[132] In response, Whitaker writes, "Fava has been banging this drum for 16 years now. One wishes that the NIMH and American psychiatry would, at long last, address this concern head-on, and inform the public about it too. But I am not holding my breath."

A 2016 study took data from an online survey of 180 people in New Zealand who had taken antidepressants long-term (3–15 years). Overall, they said they were less depressed and had a better quality of life because of the drugs, but about 30% still said they had moderate or severe depression. Many reported concerns over adverse effects; withdrawal effects (73.5%), sexual problems (71.8%), weight gain (65.3%) and adverse emotional effects; feeling emotionally numb (64.5%) and addicted (43%.) They said there needs to be more information about long-term risks.[133]

A Sky News report warned "Long-term antidepressant users are risking permanent damage to their bodies, according to leading medical experts." Tony Kendrick, a professor of primary care at the University of Southampton, said, "By the time we find out what the effects of long-term use are it may be too late to help those people, the effects could be permanent. If it does cause an increased risk of stroke or seizures or effect on the kidneys, these things may only come to light as you get older and it may be very difficult to treat those. We're seeing some of the longer-term side effects. Generally, most people are okay on them, but a few people can get bleeding from the stomach, they can get bleeding in the brain so they get strokes, they can get epileptic fits." Interestingly, Kendrick admits "scientists are not exactly sure how the antidepressants work and therefore what long-terms effects they might have."[134]

In Michael P. Hengartner's 2020 article, "How effective are antidepressants for depression over the long term? A critical review of relapse prevention trials and the issue of withdrawal confounding," he concludes, "This article concurs with a growing number of physicians and researchers who caution against indiscriminate long-term antidepressant treatment. Currently, there is no reliable evidence that long-term antidepressant treatment is beneficial and there are legitimate concerns that it may be largely ineffective or even harmful in a substantial portion of users. It is particularly problematic that we have almost no data on antidepressants' long-term effects on objective measures of social functioning (e.g. employment and disability rates) and patient-oriented outcomes such as quality of life. A critical reappraisal of current treatment guidelines along these lines is required."[135]

Possible Long-Term Effects

Chronic Brain Impairment (CBI)

Antidepressants are neurotoxic. They can harm the brain and disrupt its functions. They can produce adverse effects on the structure or function of the central and/or peripheral nervous system. Like all psychiatric drugs, antidepressants have biochemical effects and other neurotransmitter systems react to these effects and broader changes can begin to occur in the brain and in mental functioning over time.

Twenty years ago, in his 2001 paper, "Psychiatric drug induced Chronic Brain Impairment (CBI): Implications for long term treatment with Psychiatric Medication," Peter Breggin describes one long-term effect as "Chronic Brain Impairment" (CBI). He describes it as being associated with generalized brain dysfunction manifesting itself in an overall compromise of mental function. The symptoms include but are not limited to; cognitive deficits often first noticed as short-term memory dysfunction and impaired new learning difficulty with attention and concentration, apathy, indifference (or an overall loss of enjoyment and interest in life activities), affective dysregulation (including emotional lability), loss of empathy, increased irritability and finally a lack of self -awareness about these changes in mental function and behavior.[136]

He comments, "It is difficult to estimate what percentage of patients will develop CBI after years of exposure to psychiatric drugs. In my clinical experience, nearly all patients who remain on these chemical agents for many years will develop some symptoms of CBI. If the patient is taking multiple psychiatric drugs for years at a time, in my experience CBI is always marked."

Dementia

A 2016 study in Canada concluded, "Antidepressant drug usage is associated with AD/dementia and this is particularly evident if usage begins before age 65 and use of antidepressant drugs was associated with a significant twofold increase in the odds of some form of cognitive impairment or dementia."[137]

A 2018 study published in the British Medical Journal, found a "robust link" between the degenerative disease and the medication, even when taken up to 20 years before a diagnosis. It suggests some patients with long-term exposure to the drugs could face a 30 percent increased chance of dementia."[138]

Chris Fox, Professor of Clinical Psychiatry at UEA's Norwich Medical School said, "Doctors and patients should therefore be vigilant about using anticholinergic medications. It is becoming apparent we need to consider the risk of long-term cognitive effects, as well as short-term effects when we look at the benefits and risks when considering taking antidepressants."[139]

Diabetes

Studies suggest that long-term antidepressant use may be associated with an increased risk of type 2 diabetes, especially for young adults. A study in Taiwan reported; "increasing mean daily dose or use of selective serotonin reuptake inhibitors or serotonin antagonist and reuptake inhibitors was associated with increased diabetes risk."[140]

A large, population-based cohort Study in Japan looked at the "Association Between the Use of Antidepressants and the Risk of Type 2 Diabetes Mellitus." Its findings were, "Long-term antidepressant use increased the risk of type 2 diabetes onset in a time-and dose-dependent manner. Glucose tolerance improved when antidepressants were discontinued, or the dose was reduced after diabetes onset."[141]

Tardive Dysphoria

One of the most concerning potential long-term adverse effects is tardive dysphoria. It is perhaps unsurprising worsened depression caused by antidepressants has been given a medical sounding name. It's the name given to our state when the drugs might have literally worsened our depression. It is now believed there is "emerging evidence that, in some individuals, persistent use of antidepressants may be pro-depressant."[142] It can even occur in some of us who were never depressed but were perhaps prescribed an antidepressant for one of many other conditions.

It is thought the problem may be that the "oppositional tolerance" process, means we end up with a depleted serotonergic system. The postsynaptic neurons end up with a reduced density of receptors for serotonin. El-Mallakh writes that "a chronic and treatment-resistant depressive state is proposed to occur in individuals who are exposed to potent antagonists of serotonin reuptake pumps [i.e., SSRIs] for prolonged periods. Due to the delay in the onset of this chronic depressive state, it is labeled tardive dysphoria. Tardive dysphoria manifests as a chronic dysphoric state that is initially transiently relieved by—but ultimately becomes unresponsive to—antidepressant medication. Serotonergic antidepressants may be of particular importance in the development of tardive dysphoria." Robert Whitaker asks a very important question; "Many teenagers are now being prescribed an antidepressant, and when they take the drug, their brains will develop "oppositional tolerance" to it. What percentage of these youth will end up with drug-induced tardive dysphoria, and thus suffer a lifetime of chronic depression?"[143]

Treatment Resistant Depression

According to Jaskaran Singh, MD, Senior Director of Neuroscience, Janssen Pharmaceuticals, part of the Johnson & Johnson family of companies; "Although there is some disagreement as to how to define treatment-resistant depression, a patient is generally considered to have it if the individual hasn't responded to adequate doses of two different antidepressants taken for a sufficient duration of time, which is usually six weeks."[144]

They believe it exists in up to 30 percent of all patients treated with antidepressants. Along with it can come suicide ideation, self-harming, functional impairment and relapse. But haven't we heard all this somewhere before? Don't these appear in the list of adverse effects of antidepressant treatment and withdrawal effects?

"Treatment-resistant depression, a complex clinical problem caused by multiple risk factors, is targeted by integrated therapeutic strategies, which include optimization of medications, a combination of antidepressants, switching of antidepressants, and augmentation with non-antidepressants, psychosocial and cultural therapies, and somatic therapies including electroconvulsive therapy, repetitive transcranial magnetic stimulation, magnetic seizure therapy, deep brain stimulation, transcranial direct current stimulation, and vagus nerve stimulation."[145]

So, a complex clinical problem, perhaps caused by antidepressants not only requires more treatment with drugs but also other dangerous and potentially life crippling treatments such as electroconvulsive therapy (ECT). A classic example of where our initial treatment with antidepressants, for a mild and self-limiting bout of sadness, might eventually lead us.

Tolerance

The medical profession admits that another poorly understood area is why some of us report our antidepressants have stopped working, sometimes referred to as "poop out" or tachyphylaxis.

"Patients affected by ADT tachyphylaxis experience a noticeably sudden progressive decrease in response to SSRIs. The reported rates of this condition vary from 9% to 33% of SSRI users, and the majority of those affected seem to be less responsive to subsequent treatments. In most observational studies, these individuals suffer a recurrence or relapse of depression without changing the previously effective dose."[146]

So called antidepressant tolerance usually results in our doctor providing a new prescription. "When confronted with the possibility that an antidepressant may have lost its effectiveness, the clinician has one of four options. The first option, and one usually followed by most clinicians, is to increase the dose of the antidepressant, which may produce a return of effectiveness. Problems associated with this option include the emergence of side effects and increase in cost. Moreover, the improvement of most patients with this management strategy is transient so that subsequent augmentation or change to a different class of antidepressant is needed."[147]

Rather than our new "antidepressed" unbalanced/balanced state no longer working, could it be, just like the first time we were prescribed our medication, we are once again simply being human and reacting to new everyday life events the way we as humans might be expected to? It is important to remember antidepressants are not a vaccine to shield us from the trials and tribulations of everyday life. Antidepressants might help us cope with life in the short-term, but the term "tolerance" is yet one more example of a situation when we will be further medicated, dose might reach the maximum which can be prescribed, and additional drugs might be introduced leading to polypharmacy.

14
DEPENDENCE AND OUR NEW BALANCED STATE

No one knows how long it takes to become "dependent" on antidepressants but there are millions of us unaware we are.

> *Being dependent on antidepressants means we need the drugs to function physically and mentally in what has become our new "antidepressed" normal state and we need to maintain the levels of the antidepressant in our system to stay in our new "normal". Any reduction or changes to our antidepressant regimen can induce physical and mental adverse effects. The antidepressants we have taken to supposedly cure a chemical imbalance have instead created their own balanced state which, without them, it is impossible to maintain.*[148]

Dependence is not addiction. According to the National Institute on Drug Abuse (NIDA), "Addiction is defined as a chronic, relapsing disorder characterized by compulsive drug seeking, continued use despite harmful consequences, and long-lasting changes in the brain. It is considered both a complex brain disorder and a mental illness. Addiction is the most severe form of a full spectrum of substance use disorders, and is a medical illness caused by repeated misuse of a substance or substances."[149] If we are dependent, we do not crave antidepressants, there is no drug seeking behavior, urge to "use", and taking them does not usually have an effect on our ability to function socially.

No one knows exactly how long it takes to become dependent on antidepressants. There are many variables involved. Regardless of the time we have taken the drug, there is no test to show how dependent or "unbalanced" we might or might not be. The brain and body get used to the psychoactive drug and just like when we started taking it, if we reduce or stop, imbalances can occur. After taking antidepressants for a prolonged period of time we know that missing just one dose can often cause problems such as dizziness, brain zaps and feelings of sickness. It can be one of the first indications we might be dependent.

Many have taken antidepressants since the 1990s. It is important to remember that for a long time there was no online information or support groups, and what we knew about the drugs was limited. Dependence on antidepressants is now a significant public health issue as more of us become long-term users.

"Long-term use of antidepressants is surging in the United States, according to a new analysis of federal data by The New York Times. Some 15.5 million Americans have been taking the medications for at least five years. The rate has almost doubled since 2010, and more than tripled since 2000. Nearly 25 million adults have been on antidepressants for at least two years, a 60 percent increase since 2010. The drugs have helped millions of people ease depression and anxiety and are widely regarded as milestones in psychiatric treatment. Many, perhaps most people, stop the medications without significant trouble. But the rise in long time use is also the result of an unanticipated and growing problem: Many who try to quit say they cannot because of withdrawal symptoms they were never warned about."[150]

The truth is that many people find it difficult to withdraw from antidepressants because of their withdrawal symptoms caused by dependence. The more dependent we are, the more withdrawal symptoms we might suffer and the more difficult it might be for us to stop taking them.

Dependence along with lack of understanding of the issue of withdrawal and lack of knowledgeable support mean more of us are choosing to remain blissfully ignorant dependents.

The medical profession is becoming aware antidepressant dependence is an issue it needs to address but there are many confusing and mixed messages regarding antidepressant dependence. It is becoming such a problem that in the UK the British Medical Association (BMA) have recommended a number of actions be taken to help address the issue. They recognize the need for a national 24-hour helpline to support people with prescribed drug dependence. There are a handful of support services in the UK that might be able to help but the BMA is calling for a national approach to support, which would allow doctors to refer patients to support in their local area.[151]

There are millions of people who are unaware of the problems that dependence might cause them. Doctors should make us aware of possible dependence when we are considering taking antidepressants and it is one of the most important factors in our informed consent. Anecdotal evidence now tells us it probably doesn't take very long to become dependent and it is one of the main reasons, if we choose to take antidepressants, we should stay on them for the shortest time possible. As soon as we start to feel better it is time to consider reducing and withdrawing with the help of a doctor. When and if we should come off antidepressants is a personal choice requiring serious thought for serious reasons, our potential dependence being one of them.

Dependence on antidepressants can make us vulnerable.

Being vulnerable when we take antidepressants is rarely talked about. Being dependent on antidepressants can make us vulnerable for many reasons. Imagine, after years of taking a drug as prescribed, we suddenly find we are without it, unable to access it, or in a position where we are unable to communicate the vital need to have our medication. If we are without our medication we will inevitably go into involuntary withdrawal, often with horrendous consequences.

If we are uneducated and not informed about our medication, we are vulnerable. Prescribers should make us aware of the benefits and risks of antidepressants. Unfortunately, this is not always the case. It can be up to us to inform ourselves, to the best of our ability, about our need to keep ourselves as safe as we can when we take antidepressants.

This is particularly important for the elderly and those who find themselves without personal support. Having access to the drugs which have caused dependence can literally be the difference between life and death. Finding ourselves in a position where we are no longer able to make our own decisions about our medication can result in medications being both unnecessarily deprescribed or overprescribed.

A medicated child or young person will eventually move away from home and the security of their parent, care provider or local doctor/ prescriber. If they are not educated about the dangers of suddenly stopping taking their medication and their potential dependence, this might result in illness, further mental health issues or in some cases suicide.

Millions in the US don't take their medications due to the cost. Drugs can cost up to three times more than in the rest of the world.[152] With antidepressants, it is more complicated than simply "if we stop taking them, they just stop working." Skipping doses or stopping antidepressants cold turkey can be fatal. If we think we might be dependent on antidepressants, we need to regard them as essential. We cannot suddenly stop antidepressants without some risks. Being unable to afford antidepressants and where to access low-cost treatments generates much online discussion and often unreliable advice.

This is concerning, as it affects millions of Americans.

"An estimated one in 10 Americans is struggling to afford coverage and medications, and about 16 percent of Americans take a psychiatric medication. That means somewhere between 2.5 to 5 million people are having trouble accessing the psychiatric medications they need. Even under normal circumstances, such a sudden lack would be a public health crisis. But the pandemic, as Montgomery pointed out, is triggering in itself. During March, the Disaster Distress Helpline, a government-run counseling hotline, witnessed a 338 percent increase in call volume compared to February."[153]

Drug shortages can leave us vulnerable to the adverse effects of sudden discontinuation of an antidepressant or having to switch to a different antidepressant. There are already reports of patients suffering self-harm and suicidal ideation due to drug shortages. One news report from Canada writes, "The effects of the first shortage [were] extremely devastating. During that month, I had chronic suicidal ideation, I barely ate, I was unable to leave home and work. It basically compromised my whole immune system. It has cost me my income, relationships, it even sent me to the hospital because of my panic attacks."[154]

We are becoming increasingly aware helplines and charities do not understand or fail to recognize the adverse or withdrawal effects of antidepressants. They are often told not to discuss antidepressants with those who need help and ignore the fact that suddenly being without antidepressants can be a red flag warning for potential suicide. Some organizations' reliance on funding from the pharmaceutical industry has been questioned as the reason for their silence.

Antidepressant dependence needs to be regarded as a pre-existing condition; after all, it is iatrogenic harm and caused by the medication which has been legally prescribed.

15
WITHDRAWAL: THE RELAPSE TRAP AND RESEARCH

Blaming withdrawal effects on "relapse" has resulted in millions taking antidepressants long-term.

Scientific research has long suggested that the reduction or discontinuation, both gradual and abrupt, of antidepressants determines the appearance of withdrawal symptoms. Usually the patient interprets (and unfortunately also many clinicians) these symptoms as a recurrence of the disease following therapy reduction. On the contrary, this phenomenon has been described in the scientific literature as caused by the abstinence from SSRI (Selective Serotonin Reuptake Inhibitor) antidepressants or SNRI (Serotonin and Noradrenaline Reuptake Inhibitor) antidepressants.[155]

The first time we might become aware of our inability to cope without our antidepressants is probably when we miss a dose or when we begin to taper / reduce too quickly. We are probably experiencing symptoms indicating we have some degree of dependence. Doctors, however, will probably tell us our symptoms are due to "relapse" and we need our antidepressants! The terms "relapse" and "discontinuation syndrome" are convenient terms adopted by the medical profession to keep us taking our medication and as evidence we need our antidepressants.

Dr. Giovanni Fava, a leading researcher of adverse effects of antidepressants explained in *Psychiatric Times*, "If you teach a psychiatric resident that symptoms that occur during tapering cannot be due to withdrawal they are likely to interpret [the symptoms] as signs of relapse and to go back to treatment—exactly what 'Big Pharma' likes. The term "discontinuation syndrome" applied to antidepressants, versus "withdrawal syndromes" compared with benzodiazepines, was a very smart method of the pharmaceutical industry to deny the problem."[156]

We are told antidepressants prevent relapse, but Michael Hengartner writes "the argument that antidepressants are useful for preventing relapse comes "almost exclusively" from "discontinuation trials." In these studies, people who respond well to antidepressants are randomly assigned to two groups: one group remains on the drug, and the other abruptly stop taking the drug."[157]

Christopher Lane, Ph.D. author and teacher of medical humanities and the history of medicine at Northwestern University writes, "When patients try to end treatment, even stepping down their dose very gradually, many of them (22% to 78%, according to Rosenbaum and Fava[158]) find that the receptors in their serotonergic system—saturated artificially for months, even years—experience the drop to pre-drug levels as starvation. Some patients then find themselves at the mercy of hair-trigger symptoms that register as intense anxiety, aggression, and insomnia.

"As the proportion of SSRI-takers found to suffer from discontinuation syndrome is, by pharmacological standards, astronomical, and "one in 10 Americans"—roughly 30 million people in the U.S. alone—"ingests" the drugs each year, as Peter Kramer noted only last week,[159] it seems incredible that clinical trials have been so slow to recognize, and isolate for, withdrawal syndrome in patients trying to taper and end SSRI treatment. The number of people affected would, in any normal situation, drive a lot more targeted research on the problem."

However, while drug-companies have done their best to redefine withdrawal syndrome as relapse, to confuse doctors and patients into thinking the original depression or anxiety had returned, the good news is that research is starting to focus exclusively on the widespread problem of SSRI withdrawal syndrome.[160]

"When antidepressant treatment is started, future discontinuation, including the risk for relapse—as well as discontinuation symptoms—should be discussed. Based on the author's experience, this discussion seldom takes place, although it could affect patients' decisions regarding treatment options (cognitive behavior therapy vs medication)."[161]

Why is the issue of antidepressant withdrawal, hardly ever discussed when we are first prescribed antidepressants? Do prescribers purposely avoid the issue they seem to know so little about or do they think if we were initially told about withdrawal symptoms we might think differently about taking them?

It would be very rare for antidepressant withdrawal symptoms to be exactly the same as the original symptoms we were suffering when we received our initial prescription. If we think about why we first started taking antidepressants, what was happening in our life then and how we felt, it is probably pretty easy to see that missing a few doses of antidepressants or a failed attempt at withdrawal is not a relapse. How can we suddenly have miraculously returned to our original or a similar "condition?" It is very common for doctors to tell us it is a return of our original problems or another episode of depression. This in turn often leads to long-term treatment with antidepressants.

Not advising patients when they are first prescribed antidepressants of the potential difficulty they might have withdrawing has perhaps led to the unnecessary medication of millions. It is one of the most important discussions needed to enable real informed consent. Blaming adverse effects or withdrawal effects on relapse or discontinuation syndrome has meant millions of us have been persuaded to remain on antidepressants longer than needed. It has also delayed crucial research being undertaken to develop withdrawal guidelines and protocols. As Christopher Lane says, "The number of people affected would, in any normal situation, drive a lot more targeted research on the problem," but this is not a normal situation. Once again, it is all about the power of the pharmaceutical marketing language used in their strategy to keep us medicated.

What research has been done to look at antidepressant withdrawal effects and why has this area been neglected?

Although the first antidepressant, Prozac, was introduced in 1988, the first systematic review on withdrawal was not published until 2015. There were almost 200 meta-analyses on the efficacy of new-generation antidepressants published between 2007 and 2014. Most of these efficacy studies were pharmaceutical funded at a time when they were trying to prove to each other, "our antidepressant is better than your antidepressant."

When it first became apparent some of us were having difficulty withdrawing from antidepressants, the pharmaceutical industry adopted the term "discontinuation syndrome," rather than withdrawal effects to try to cover up the severity of problems we were encountering.

Massabki and Abi-Jaoude write, "From a critical review of the term discontinuation syndrome in the literature, it is clear that the use of the term in place of withdrawal is not justified... the use of the term in the literature grew markedly after pharmaceutical company– sponsored conferences in 1997 and 2006. The term discontinuation syndrome, compared with its counterpart withdrawal, does not entail similar negative connotation and, as a result, may serve to reduce patients' fears of dependence. Several authors have expressed concerns that if patients worry about developing dependence or addiction to antidepressants, they may decide to not pursue such treatments. Such arguments are inconsistent with principles of autonomy and informed consent. An aforementioned survey of 1829 individuals taking antidepressants found that only 1% recalled having been informed about withdrawal effects when they were prescribed the drug. The use of the term withdrawal better enables patients to make appropriately informed decisions."[162]

In the 2018 review, "A systematic review into the incidence, severity and duration of antidepressant withdrawal effects: Are guidelines evidence-based?" Dr. James Davies and Professor John Read questioned the UK's current National Institute for Health and Care Excellence (NICE) and the American Psychiatric Association's (APA) depression guidelines, which said withdrawal reactions from antidepressants are "self-limiting" (i.e. typically resolving between 1 and 2 weeks). Davies and Read conducted a literature review to better understand the incidence, severity and duration of antidepressant withdrawal reactions.

They identified 23 relevant studies, with different methodologies and sample sizes and concluded "More than half (56%) of people who attempt to come off antidepressants experience withdrawal effects. Nearly half (46%) of people experiencing withdrawal effects describe them as severe. It is not uncommon for the withdrawal effects to last for several weeks or months. Current UK and USA Guidelines underestimate the severity and duration of antidepressant withdrawal, with significant clinical implications.

We recommend that UK and USA guidelines on antidepressant withdrawal be urgently updated as they are clearly at variance with the evidence on the incidence, severity, and duration of antidepressant withdrawal, and are probably leading to the widespread misdiagnosing of withdrawal, the consequent lengthening of antidepressant use, much unnecessary antidepressant prescribing and higher rates of antidepressant prescriptions overall. We also recommend that prescribers fully inform patients about the possibility of withdrawal effects."[163]

What we actually do know about antidepressant withdrawal effects comes mostly from the experiences of patients and anecdotal evidence. It is not through scientific research but through listening to the experiences of others, mostly online. Thankfully, scientific literature is now starting to agree with patient experiences and in "Withdrawal-the tide is finally turning,"[164,165] Michael P. Hengartner, John Read and James Davies write about the progress made when making the case that withdrawal from antidepressant drugs is often longer-lasting and severe.

"Withdrawal reactions when coming off antidepressants have long been neglected or minimized. It took almost two decades after the selective serotonin reuptake inhibitors (SSRIs) entered the market for the first systematic review to be published. More reviews have followed, demonstrating that the dominant and long-held view that withdrawal is mostly mild, affects only a small minority and resolves spontaneously within 1–2 weeks, was at odds with the sparse but growing evidence base. What the scientific literature reveals is in close agreement with the thousands of service user testimonies available online in large forums. It suggests that withdrawal reactions are quite common, that they may last from a few weeks to several months or even longer, and that they are often severe. These findings are now increasingly acknowledged by official professional bodies and societies."[166,167]

Once again, the point is made that if we knew about the seriousness of withdrawal effects, many of us would choose not to take antidepressants or would limit the time we take them. They highlight the lack of support and the fact that we are often told that withdrawal symptoms are due to the return of our illness. Thanks to Davies and Read and the many campaigners in the UK, the National Institute for Health and Care Excellence (NICE), amended its 2009 guidelines on depression to recognize the severity and length of antidepressant withdrawal symptoms. The new guidelines state that withdrawal symptoms may be severe and protracted in some patients.

For some, fear of withdrawal symptoms is often the reason so many patients take antidepressants for long periods. Some doctors still choose to deny our symptoms are those of withdrawal and just as with adverse effects, it is not uncommon for patients to be ignored when complaining about withdrawal symptoms. There is still so much misinformation online about withdrawal symptoms, why we have them, how long they last and how to prevent them.

Recognizing withdrawal effects is one issue but how to prevent them happening is surely the one we now need to address. We urgently need to have official guidelines on how to help prevent harm and ensure we can manage antidepressant withdrawal safely. It is at this point we need to be reminded just how "wicked" a problem this is.[168]

What are the symptoms we might experience when withdrawing from antidepressants?

The Inner Compass Initiative's "The Withdrawal Project" sums up withdrawal effects perfectly when it describes them as "unique". They can be varied and unpredictable and different for every one of us.

"Another by-product of psychiatric drug-induced dependence is the emergence of mental, emotional, physical, cognitive, and sleep-related problems upon the reduction or cessation of a medication. Psychiatric drug withdrawal is a very unique, individual experience that can involve few or many of a vast spectrum of symptoms. It is becoming clear based on anecdotal reports from the withdrawal community that two people can take the same amount of the same drug or take a drug for the same length of time and have completely different withdrawal experiences."[169]

Some of the most common withdrawal effects reported; headaches, electric shock sensations (e.g. "brain zaps"), paresthesia or burning, prickly or skin-crawling sensations, flu-like symptoms, nausea, tiredness, insomnia and sleep issues, dizziness and vertigo, vivid dreams, nightmares, amnesia, irritability, nervousness and anxiety, panic attacks, depersonalization, agitation and depression, mania, aggressive or impulsive behavior, suicidal ideation, akathisia, psychosis, cognitive impairment, mood problems, excessive sweating, sexual dysfunction, gastrointestinal issues, movement disorders, speech changes, sensory problems like tinnitus, drop in blood pressure, muscle pain or weakness.

We know withdrawal effects are more likely with higher doses of antidepressants or/and the longer our exposure to the medication. Antidepressants with shorter half-lives are likely to produce more effects and within a shorter period of time (2 days as opposed 2-6 weeks for antidepressants with a longer half-life). The half-life of an antidepressant is the time it takes for our body to break down and remove half of a medication from our system.

An antidepressant with a short half-life leaves our body faster than one with a longer half-life.

Antidepressant	Approximate Half-Life (Hours)
Citalopram	36
Desvenlafaxine	11
Duloxetine	30
Escitalopram	8–17

Antidepressant	Approximate Half-Life (Hours)
Fluoxetine	96–144
Fluvoxamine	24
Levomilnacipran	12
Milnacipran	8
Paroxetine	17–22
Sertraline	22–36
Venlafaxine	4–7

What does the existing research tell us about the best way to withdraw from antidepressants?

> *"About 37 million in the US are prescribed antidepressants in any given month (about 13% of the adult population) and half of those have been taking them for at least 5 years. We now know for certain that millions of people in the US and beyond struggle when they try to come off these drugs. Underestimating the problem is not going to help patients get the accurate information, and the withdrawal support services, they need and deserve."*[170]

Very little research has been done regarding how to withdraw from antidepressants. This is because the medical profession has denied the severity of withdrawal effects and how difficult it can be to stop taking them. They have preferred to remain uneducated and accepting of the fact that the easiest (and most profitable) option is to keep prescribing and keep us medicated.

In their most recent Guideline on Major Depressive Disorder, in 2010, the American Psychiatric Association write, "When pharmacotherapy is being discontinued, it is best to taper the medication over the course of at least several weeks. Such tapering allows for the detection of recurring symptoms at a time when patients are still partially treated and therefore more easily returned to full therapeutic treatment if needed. In addition, such tapering can help minimize the incidence of antidepressant medication discontinuation syndromes, particularly with paroxetine and venlafaxine."

The UK Royal College of Psychiatry leaflet, "Stopping Antidepressants", which was published in 2020, tells us, "This is different for everyone. If you have been taking an antidepressant for only a few weeks you may be able to reduce, and stop, over a month or so. Even if you have only mild (or no) withdrawal symptoms, it is best to do this over at least four weeks. If you have been taking antidepressants for many months or years, it's best to taper more slowly (again, at a rate you find comfortable). This will usually be over a period of months or longer. It's also best to reduce the dose slowly if you have had withdrawal symptoms in the past."

But on what research are these inadequate guidelines from two incredibly powerful and respected organizations based on? Where are the worldwide studies to help the millions trying to withdraw from antidepressants?

In their 2019 paper, "Tapering of SSRI treatment to mitigate withdrawal symptoms."[171] Dr. Mark Horowitz, PhD, and Professor David Taylor recommend hyperbolic tapering. "SSRIs work by inhibiting the serotonin transporter, and the relationship between the dose and the level of binding to the transporter is hyperbolic. When the patient is taking low doses, the level of binding increases very rapidly, and then levels off at higher doses. A patient using only registered doses takes steps down which are too large. When the patient begins tapering from a high dose, these steps have a limited impact on transporter binding. But, at low doses, this impact is significant.

So, even a small dose decrease can have a big effect. This hyperbolic relationship explains why withdrawal symptoms are often most problematic towards the end of a taper. Dose steps down that are lower than registered doses are required to achieve smaller steps to avoid withdrawal symptoms—this is known as hyperbolic tapering."[172]

"We suggest that, in the absence of more robust evidence to guide tapering (especially where guidelines advise to taper gradually without specific instructions), the tapering regimen described here should be considered for adoption into clinical practice. There are few disadvantages of recommending slower tapers. It should at least be recognized that tapering periods of 2–4 weeks are likely to be inadequate for reducing withdrawal symptoms for many patients, with longer periods of tapering, and regimens that include lower doses of medication, more likely to be effective. Further empirical study of tapering regimens, including the one proposed here, is urgently required, with a consequent update of formal guidelines."[173]

In April 2021, in the Cochrane Report "Approaches for discontinuation versus continuation of long-term antidepressant use for depressive and anxiety disorders in adults", Dr Mark Horowitz and Belgian-based researcher and GP, Dr Ellen Van Leeuwen, looked at the findings from 33 Random Controlled Trials (RCTs) that included 4,995 participants who were prescribed antidepressants for 24 weeks or longer. In 13 studies, the antidepressant was stopped abruptly; in 18, it was stopped over a few weeks (known as 'tapering'); in four, psychological therapy support was also offered; and in one study, stopping was prompted by a letter to GPs with guidance on tapering. Most tapering schemes lasted four weeks or less and none of the studies used very slow tapering schemes beyond a few weeks - in contrast to new guidelines from the UK Royal College of Psychiatrists that recommend tapering over months or years to safely stop.

"We compared different approaches and looked at benefits (such as successful stopping rates) and harms (such as return of the depressive or anxiety episodes, side effects and withdrawal symptoms)," says Dr Van Leeuwen. "Our review outlines detailed findings across all these areas, but in a nutshell there was only very low certainty evidence on the pros and cons of each of the different approaches to stopping—making it difficult to reach any firm conclusions at this time. The key issue is that studies do not distinguish between symptoms of a return (or relapse) of depression and symptoms of withdrawal after stopping, and that's really problematic."

In "Strategies to reduce use of antidepressants",[174] Professor Tony Kendrick suggests, "Prescribers should actively review long-term antidepressant use and suggest coming off them slowly to patients who are well. The relationship between SSRI dose and serotonin transporter receptor occupancy suggests that hyperbolic tapering regimes may be helpful for patients with troubling withdrawal symptoms who cannot stop treatment within 4–8 weeks, and tapering strips can allow carefully titrated slower dose reduction over some months. Internet and telephone support to patients wanting to reduce their antidepressants is being trialed in the REDUCE programme." The REDUCE Programme[175] is a UK £2.4 million funded 6-year project (2016-2022); "We aim to identify feasible, safe, reliable and cost-effective (value for money) ways of helping patients withdraw from long-term antidepressants, where this is appropriate."[176]

In Australia, a trial called STOPS[177] (STructured Online intervention to Promote and Support antidepressant de-prescribing in primary care), is aiming to provide on-line guidance (called WiserAd) and practice nurse support to patients. "The incidence of antidepressant withdrawal symptoms in representative samples of patients tapering off antidepressants and risk factors which predict more withdrawal symptoms in prospective studies to avoid recall bias" are also being studied by the OPERA project,[178] a Netherlands Study of Optimal, PERsonal Antidepressant use.

Much more research and larger trials on how to safely withdraw from antidepressants are urgently needed to compare different tapering methods. We urgently need the pharmaceutical industry to produce drugs in lower doses and as liquid formulation. We need official and evidence-based guidelines to educate professionals and the public on how to safely manage their antidepressants, but one thing is very clear, there will never be one single solution to this growing problem. Because of the many variables, it seems there might only ever be guidelines. We now recognize withdrawal effects can sometimes be severe, but we are still presented with solving the problem of how to stop taking antidepressants and preventing possible harm.

Is it time to ask who the real experts are? We are realizing the medical profession has, for the foreseeable future, no good answers for people struggling to stop taking antidepressants and no means to determine who is at highest risk of being unable to stop. It is time to face the fact that if anything is going to change, it will be because of the valuable and substantial existing and growing patient experiences and their knowledge. As governments and the medical profession continue to underestimate and ignore the problem, we find ourselves in a situation where, for the current time at least, it is down to the power of patient experience to change and improve the situation we find ourselves in.

Tapering strips might enable us to have more control of our antidepressant reductions.

One of the difficulties when trying to withdraw or reduce antidepressants is they only come in a limited number of doses. Making very small reductions can be difficult and we often need to resort to cutting pills, counting beads or taking a liquid if available. Tapering strips are 28-day rolls of daily pouches of antidepressants. They can be used to reduce our antidepressant doses at a rate decided by us. They enable us to make much smaller dose reductions so we can work with our prescriber to create a personalized tapering schedule at a much slower rate. The key is to avoid large cuts in dose to minimize withdrawal effects. This enables a hyperbolic taper with smaller and smaller doses, as recommended by Mark Horowitz and David Taylor.[179]

"Tapering strips allow patients to regulate the tempo of their dose reduction over time and enable them to taper more gradually, conveniently and safely than is possible using currently available standard medication, thereby preventing withdrawal symptoms."[180]

The evidence says they work. In a recent study "The previously reported 71% short-term success rate of tapering strips in the most severely affected group, was matched by a 68% rate after 1–5 years. The evidence-based approach of personal tapering to counter withdrawal, as used for drugs causing withdrawal, for example, benzodiazepines, may represent a simple solution for an important antidepressant-related public health problem, without extra costs."[181]

The Tapering Project was established in 2010 to develop tapered doses of medication and tapering strips are available in the Netherlands.[182] They can be sent worldwide (legislation allowing). They are available for a wide range of drugs including antipsychotics and sedatives. There is an obvious need for the pharmaceutical industry to make antidepressants available in lower doses or, in an ideal world, produce tapering strips themselves.

A petition in the UK is asking the UK medical authorities to trial and implement tapering strips which provide the most commonly prescribed medications in decreasing doses over a period of time. It is hoped this will help millions of users of psychoactive prescription drugs. This petition can be found at https//www.change.org/p/provide-tapering-strips-to-help-people-withdraw-from-antidepressant-and-antipsychotic-drugs.

PART 3

Safe Antidepressant Management and Withdrawal

16

ADOPTING A HARM REDUCTION APPROACH

There are many reasons it is important we never stop taking or start withdrawing from antidepressants or other psychotropic medication without the support of a knowledgeable medical professional or support service. Antidepressant treatment should be supported by frequent reviews. We need to be aware, from the very first pill we take, of any physical or psychological changes we experience and report them immediately to our prescriber. Evidence suggests the risk of suicide, self-harm or other severe adverse events is significantly higher when commencing, stopping or changing doses or switching drugs including generics.

When should we consider "coming off" or managing our antidepressants?

The simple answer is if we decide to take antidepressants, we should stay on them for the shortest time possible. If we were told when we were given our very first prescription that stopping taking antidepressants can be incredibly difficult and even dangerous for some, it might have made us think twice about our choices. Being told this rarely happens and for many of us, it is not until we are faced with the challenge of reducing antidepressants, we realize how little we know about the psychoactive drug we might have ingested for years or sometimes decades. It is often at this time we realize the significant effects antidepressants have had on our minds and bodies.

In an article published in the British Journal of General Practice, (BJGP), researcher and campaigner Stevie Lewis writes about her experience with antidepressant withdrawal. In "The four research papers I wish my doctor had read before prescribing an antidepressant," she points to four significant studies that she wishes her doctor had read before prescribing her antidepressants in 1996. She goes on to summarize the findings of these important studies (found at bjgp.org/content/71/708/316/tab-article-info).

Deciding to reduce antidepressants is a personal choice. Whether or not it is right for us to stay on or try to reduce antidepressants should ALWAYS be a decision we make with the support of a knowledgeable medical professional or support service.

What are the main reasons people decide to "stop" taking antidepressants?

There are many reasons we might decide we want to stop taking antidepressants and they will be personal to us. They might include:

- Adverse effects such as lack of emotion, feeling numb, feeling tired, weight gain, depersonalization, being angry or irritable or any of the many other, sometimes serious adverse effects we can experience
- Sexual problems
- Financial reasons
- Pregnancy
- Stigma
- Feeling suicidal
- We don't think they are working, or we don't think we need them anymore

No one can tell us how our attempt to reduce antidepressants will affect us, but there are important things we need to know before start. It is about how we approach it!

Suddenly deciding to come off antidepressants is like suddenly getting up one day, and out of the blue, with no training, deciding to run a marathon. You can't do it without being prepared. Some of us, no matter how hard we train, will never run those 26 miles but might benefit substantially from being able to do a regular 5-mile walk.

We need to start by being the most informed we can be.

Just as we should when starting antidepressants, we should make informed choices about how we manage our reductions.

It is important to realize there are no tried, tested and approved ways to withdraw from antidepressants. There is so much information and guidance on the internet, but it can be difficult to work out where to start. How do we know what is the good advice and which might be harmful? We need to trust ourselves during this process and we might do well to learn about adopting an informed "Harm Reduction" approach.

"Harm Reduction is different: pragmatic, not dogmatic. Harm reduction is an international movement in community health education that recognizes there is no single solution for each person, no universal standard of "success or failure". Getting rid of the problem is not necessarily the only way. Instead, harm reduction accepts where people are at and educates them to make informed choices and calculated trade-offs that reduce risk and increase wellness. People need information, options, resources and support so they can move towards healthier living—at their own pace and on their own terms."[183]

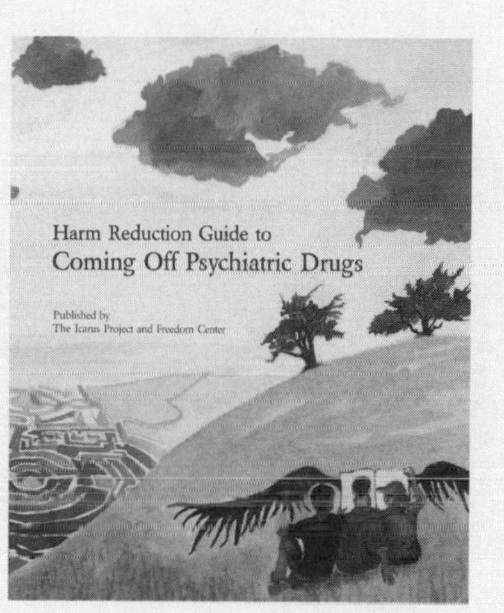

As well as the "Harm Reduction Guide" by the Icarus Project,[184] The Inner Compass Initiative have an excellent booklet to help us learn more about antidepressants and management/withdrawal.[185]

17
LEARNING ABOUT OUR ANTIDEPRESSANTS AND LISTENING TO OUR BODY

We need to learn as much as we can about the antidepressant we are taking. The Inner Compass Withdrawal Project recommends:

- "Get informed about the drugs you take
- Determine whether the medications you're planning to reduce or come off are in a 'taper-friendly' form
- Learn about risky interactions, reactions and sensitivities that can happen during withdrawal
- Review the taper rates, schedules, and methods commonly used in the layperson withdrawal community
- Walk through the various decisions, gear, and skills needed for your chosen taper method
- Get a sense of how laypeople typically implement their taper methods"[186]

Reading guidelines and patient experiences are important. Use this book's "Resource Guide" to help find guidance and reliable information.

We need to get as much support as we can.

We are advised to only take advice from a knowledgeable clinician or specialist support service but there is very little good professional support available for those of us who wish to reduce our antidepressants. Free services should be available to everyone who needs them but only a handful exist.

It is important we inform a relative, friend or colleague we trust, of our plans to reduce our medication and ask them if they will learn with us. Sometimes it is also about creating our own support system.

What if my prescriber won't support me?

Ask them to explain their reasons. They might be ones we need to consider. Let them know we are / intend to be informed and educated about the risks associated. Many people do reduce their medication without their prescriber's support, but it is always advisable to try to get them on our side.

Explain what we have read and why we think it is the best decision for us. It might be good to make them aware we realize it might be a long process and we know it doesn't have to be an all or nothing result. We should emphasize our wish to improve our health by trying to manage our medication. No one can make us take antidepressants and no one can prevent us attempting to reduce them. We need to find a professional who is willing to listen, work with us and let us choose our own rates of reductions.

Accept not all of us will be able to 'come off' antidepressants. Think about achieving that 5k walk and we might, in time, run that marathon.

The longer we have taken antidepressants, the more difficult it might be to stop taking them. If we have taken them for a long time, years rather than months, we need to go incredibly slowly. Time is our best friend, and we need to think of this in terms of a project which might take years rather than months. We also need to consider that coming off antidepressants is not always the best option for us, and our unique situation must always be considered. Not everyone will be able to come off their antidepressants successfully.

Dr. Stuart Shipko writes, "advise caution and warn of possible serious withdrawal symptoms for people with a cumulative use of antidepressants for five years or more. With cumulative use of ten years or more, I advise that there is a meaningful chance of disabling and persistent symptoms and usually do not support even attempting to taper and stop the drugs."[187]

But not everyone will find "coming off" antidepressants problematic. The shorter the time we have taken antidepressants and the lower the dose, the less problems we might have reducing them. This is not a reason to take chances with coming off too quickly and we should never quit suddenly or cold turkey unless there is a clinical reason for doing so as advised by a clinician.

Everyone starts from a different place. From the beginning we need to accept withdrawing from antidepressants cannot be "prescriptive".

It might have started with prescribing, but antidepressant withdrawal cannot be prescriptive. There is no way anyone can give us an exact personal method and timescale. It is about listening to and learning from our own body. Our particular experience with antidepressants is unique to us. We are the only one who knows our body and how it is feeling. We cannot predict how our body will react to medication reductions, but we can listen to our body and make decisions based on staying well and maintaining a quality of life. Our body will tell us if we are getting it right. We need to stay as physically and mentally balanced as we can and manage our antidepressant reductions with as few adverse effects as possible. Staying in control with the help of our professional and personal support system is vital.

It is important that we start in a balanced place. It needs to be one as free from personal, emotional and social stresses as possible. Attempting to reduce antidepressants is not the time to address the "why me?" or "who do I blame?" questions which we might have about our life on antidepressants. From the start it is important we try to remain aware of and connected to life around us. We need to keep a record of our medication reductions and any emotional and physical changes from the very start but at the same time it is important the issue does not take over our life. Being obsessed and having our lives dominated by the issue can be counterproductive.

We need to listen to our body for warnings signs we might be reducing too fast! It will tell us if our "slow" is not slow enough. "It is my strong view that for the time being it is most helpful to leave aside all sorts of theoretical considerations and agree that the most helpful approach for helping patients is to listen to them and to allow them to taper at a speed they agree with."[188]

Again, we need to keep a record of our medication reductions and any emotional and physical changes we experience. Our physical and psychological responses to dose reductions best dictates our schedule to reduce medication but it is not just about doses. It is also about making reductions at the right time.

It is important to remember that we do not know our level of dependence on antidepressants before we start this process! Severe symptoms in the early stages might indicate a higher level of dependence. This should be a warning that we need to make very small reductions very slowly. Time and patience are our best friends when it comes to reducing antidepressants. We need to try to do it with as few "withdrawal symptoms" as possible, enabling us to get on with our lives as best we can. Each time we make a reduction, our brain and body are adjusting to yet more changes and we need to give them time to adapt. Most people talk in terms of "months" for withdrawal, but anecdotal evidence tells us "years" might be needed to reduce successfully and without symptoms which impact our life. Quality of life, whilst trying to reduce, is one of the most important considerations.

Again, our response to reductions best indicates how slowly we need to reduce taking our antidepressants and warns us if we are going too fast! When we begin, because we have no idea of our level of dependence on antidepressants and it is impossible to know if our slow will be slow enough.

"Many people—especially those who taper slowly and follow careful tapering protocols in line with the messages of the body– experience few or none of these symptoms; however, many do experience at least some of them."[189]

Reducing doses incredibly slowly allows the brain and body to adapt and get used to the changes. There is no word to describe what this "slowly" really means. Patience is our best friend during this process. What is the point in wasting years tapering quickly, going back on a higher dose, constantly suffering withdrawal symptoms, if a "tortoise-like-taper" might allow us to maintain a reasonable quality of life?

Trying to reduce our antidepressants might be one of the hardest things we ever do. Readjusting and resetting involves important "rebalancing" acts, and this should never be regarded as failure.

There is little point trying to suffer and put up with "adverse effects"; with medical supervision, we can go back to the last place/dose we felt well enough to live our lives without adverse effects. If we are advised by our doctor to go back to a previous dose, this should not be regarded as a set-back but rather good and sensible medication management. We can try to make a smaller reduction next time or give ourselves much longer to get used to the previous dose. Once again, it is about listening to our body.

Beware of the "relapse" trap... we might have just gone too quickly.

Withdrawal symptoms can sometimes resemble symptoms associated with "mental illness". It is common for doctors and psychiatrists to call this relapse and prescribe us more drugs. As we have previously learned, blaming withdrawal effects on relapse has meant millions of patients have been persuaded to remain on antidepressants longer than needed. Once again this is a time to take advice, reset, slow down and maybe go back to a place we were balanced.

We have to learn to deal with normal emotions as well as dealing with the impact the drug has had on our lives. Managing and reducing antidepressants is a huge deal in anyone's life but it is important it doesn't become all consuming. We need to try to still have a life while we deal with it. It is also important not to blame every emotion we might experience on the antidepressant reduction. We should still be aware of life around us and its ups and downs. Actually, making life changes can be a useful way to focus on "living" and taking our minds off the drugs.

Be prepared to make useful life changes.

It is about looking after ourselves the best we can. Having a strong immune system is helpful. Drinking plenty of water, eating as healthily as we can and trying to exercise are important parts of the withdrawal process. More than this they can provide an outlet. We need to try to keep life as normal as possible and try to stay in control. Finding a therapist who understands the issue can also be a huge help.

Counselling and Talk Therapy

A therapist can be the human contact we need whilst we are trying to withdraw from antidepressants. The problem is finding one who understands the issues we are dealing with and also many of us are not in a position to access or pay for private therapy. Finding a therapist who understands can be a huge help. The "Guidance for Psychological Therapists" is available online and was produced by the UK All-Party Parliamentary Group for Prescribed Drug Dependence (APPG for PDD),[190] professional bodies for psychological therapists in the UK, key academics and other professionals. It aims to "support therapists in deepening their knowledge and reflection on working with clients prescribed psychiatric drugs such as antidepressants and antipsychotics."

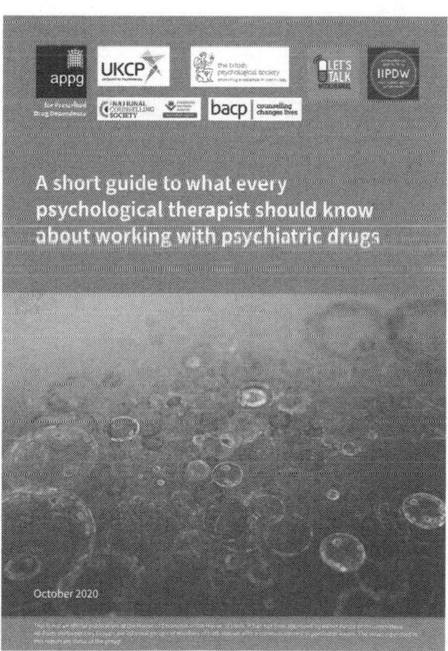

Learning the Language of Antidepressant Management and Withdrawal

The Resource Guide starting on page 246 includes websites and literature which can help us learn more about and where to find the key information we need when considering managing or withdrawing from our antidepressants. This is rarely a straightforward process, and being as knowledgeable as we can be is a powerful asset. Also included in the guide are links to published withdrawal protocols. It is important to remember we can become our own expert and should use these as guidelines not individual prescriptions. This is information and not individual advice.

18
WITHDRAWAL AND THE EXISTING PROFESSIONAL ADVICE

What "official" advice exists about withdrawing from antidepressants?

According to the New York Times analysis of federal data, "More than 15 million Americans have taken the medications for at least five years, a rate that has almost more than tripled since 2000."[191] It says, "Thousands, perhaps millions, of people who try to quit antidepressant drugs experience stinging withdrawal symptoms that last for months to years: insomnia, surges of anxiety, even so-called brain zaps, sensations of electric shock in the brain. But doctors have dismissed or downplayed such symptoms, often attributing them to the recurrence of underlying mood problems."

So where do the millions in the US and around the world go to get help? Despite perhaps millions struggling with withdrawal, the American Psychiatric Association appear to have very little to say on the issue. Their "Practice Guideline for the Treatment of Patients with Major Depressive Disorder" has not been updated since 2010. The guideline has 158 pages and on page 59, hidden in the small print, is the following brief advice on antidepressant discontinuation. "When pharmacotherapy is being discontinued, it is best to taper the medication over the course of at least several weeks. Such tapering allows for the detection of recurring symptoms at a time when patients are still partially treated and therefore more easily returned to full therapeutic treatment if needed. In addition, such tapering can help minimize the incidence of antidepressant medication discontinuation syndromes, particularly with paroxetine and venlafaxine."[192]

The APA advice is grossly inadequate, outdated and misleading. Millions of people, including our prescribers, need up to date, best practice advice and guidelines. Is this the best the American Psychiatric Association has to offer at a time when the medical profession is becoming increasingly aware this is a public health issue it urgently needs to address? Truth is, finding help withdrawing from antidepressants can prove difficult and there is little official support available.

The UK's National Institute for Health and Care Excellence's (NICE) guideline on the recognition and management of depression in adults, published in 2009, recommended that patients are tapered off their drugs over a period of up to four weeks and symptoms were "usually mild and self-limiting over about one week." Thankfully in September 2019, NICE amended its guidance to recognize that withdrawal symptoms can persist for months or more and be "more severe for some patients". The UK Royal College of Psychiatry (RCPsych) said it wanted to see a greater focus on how to help patients who are withdrawing from antidepressants and it wanted NICE to develop "clear evidence-based and pharmacologically-informed recommendations to help guide gradual withdrawal from antidepressant use." It also said it wants to see routine monitoring of when and why patients are prescribed antidepressants, and GPs being allowed the time needed to regularly review medication with patients and offer them support and advice.

In 2020, the Royal College of Psychiatrists published a leaflet on "Stopping Antidepressants".[193] This came after years of pressure from academics and campaigners who have challenged RCPscyh's previous position on antidepressant withdrawal.

The RCPysch leaflet (see the Resource Guide on page 246) comes with a disclaimer which makes it clear the "Stopping Antidepressants" leaflet provides information and not advice. RCPsych make no guarantees their content is accurate, complete or up to date. It cannot be relied on, and we need "relevant professional or specialist advice."

Undoubtedly, it is time for the developed world to address the issue of antidepressant withdrawal as a matter of urgency. It should of course be the responsibility of those who created the problem to solve it. But right now, it seems change will come from the patients and those who advocate for change. By becoming informed, educated, and sharing our knowledge, it is hoped that we will eventually reduce the role and impact antidepressants have on our lives and society.

Where do we go to find the "relevant and specialist" advice the UK Royal College of Psychiatrists suggests we take? Why do we need to be careful where we look for help?

Throughout the "Stopping Antidepressants" leaflet, we are directed to our doctor (prescriber), and pharmacist to put together our "tapering plan". Some prescribers might have the knowledge to support us, but it is generally acknowledged, prescribers urgently need education, resources and development of best practice guidelines to help their patients. The British Medical Association (BMA) has said for a number of years, "This represents a significant public health issue, one that is central to doctors' clinical role, and one that the medical profession has a clear responsibility to help address."[194] This is true throughout the developed world.

Wherever we live, it can be difficult to get reliable and knowledgeable support from the medical profession to help us manage and withdraw from antidepressants. This has left people turning to the internet for support and guidance and many informative and valuable websites have been developed. In this book's Resource Guide are the best sources of information if we want to learn the safest way to withdraw from antidepressants. They provide guidelines but we should always remember this is not personal advice.

The internet can be our best friend and our worst enemy. It requires an open-minded approach and the realization, when it comes to antidepressants, we can't trust everything we read online.

"A study of websites offering advice about antidepressants has found widespread misinformation, and widespread backing by drug companies. As people are flocking in record numbers to get their medical advice online, thanks to the coronavirus, it is time to expose the risks."[195]

Prof Peter Gøtzsche and Dr. Mayanne Demasi analyzed 39 websites published by government bodies, consumer organizations and patient advocacy groups, focusing on SSRI antidepressants, to find out how online information about the benefits and harms of medicines were being conveyed to the public.[196] All 39 websites mentioned the benefits of antidepressants. Gøtzsche and Demasi concluded, "None of the websites met our predefined criteria. The information was generally inaccurate and unhelpful and has potential to lead to inappropriate use and overuse of antidepressants and reduce the likelihood that people will seek better options for depression like psychotherapy." Twenty-nine (74%) websites attributed depression to a "chemical imbalance" or claimed they could fix an imbalance.

Sexual dysfunction was mentioned as a harmful effect on 23 (59%) websites while five (13%) mentioned emotional numbing. Twenty-five (64%) stated that antidepressants may cause increased suicidal ideation, but 23 (92%) of them contained incorrect information, and only two (5%) websites noted that the suicide risk is increased in people of all ages. Twenty-eight websites (72%) warned patients about withdrawal effects but only one stated that antidepressants can be addictive."

Many websites and forums about antidepressants have been developed and are mostly found on social media. Some of them can be excellent reliable ways to learn about all aspects of taking and withdrawing from antidepressants. Some of the sites have tens of thousands of followers. There are many debates and questions about whether Social Networking sites are good or bad for our mental health in general. People often say these sites saved their lives at a time when they could find no answers from the medical profession and yet others have warned of bullying and misinformation. One thing seems certain, at a time when many of us might feel isolated and vulnerable, social media sites can give us social support and connectedness. They can, through our self-education, give us a sense of empowerment over our situation. At the same time, it is important we remember that the evidence we find on sites is mostly anecdotal and although it can be valuable, information should be used as guidelines and not personal advice.

Online we can also find private centers, like American Addictions Centers, which talk of "Detox and Withdrawal from Antidepressants" and urge us "don't wait call us now".[197] There are "Rehab Residences" in the US where we can pay to get help. There are plenty of private clinics ready and waiting to relieve us of tens of thousands of dollars to "get off" antidepressants in what are often described as relaxing, luxurious surroundings where we will be able to "get off" antidepressants in a comfortable setting! They often promote outrageous claims such as "investigative work can begin that can isolate the factors that need to be brought in balance." Residential clinics cannot solve our antidepressant problem in a matter of weeks, and we need to be wary of their limitations and often overly optimistic promises which can come at an incredibly high financial cost. These clinics are generally alcohol and illicit drug rehabilitation services and mostly unsuitable for those who need help with antidepressants and other psychiatric medications.

"If I thought that it was possible, I would have opened a string of clinics all over the country to help get people off of antidepressants. Unfortunately, the problems that sometimes occur when people try to stop an SSRI antidepressant are much more severe and long-lasting than the medical profession acknowledges, and there is no antidote to these problems," says Stuart Shipko.[198]

PART 4

Special Concerns

19
SAME BUT NOT THE SAME: UNDERSTANDING GENERICS

Could "same but not the same" generic antidepressants be adding to the problems of antidepressant harm and dependence? In an age of consumer choice, is, "You get what you are given" acceptable?

Antidepressants have brand names and a generic name (the medical name of the drug). Generic drugs, using the medical name, can only be manufactured after the brand name drug's patent has expired. This can be up to 20 years after the patent holder's drug is first filed with the FDA. When patents or other periods of exclusivity expire, other manufacturers can submit an Abbreviated New Drug Application (ANDA) to the FDA for approval to market a generic version of the brand name drug. As an example, manufacturers were able to apply to make a generic version of sertraline in June 2006, when the patent for the brand name Zoloft expired.

We are told all manufacturers' versions of sertraline are the same as Zoloft and each other. The generic versions all contain the same mgs of sertraline, however, the differences are where they are made, size, shape, color and most importantly price. Generics can cost 20–90% less than the original price of their brand name equivalents. Unlike the brand name drug, generic sertraline is approved only on the basis of similarity and no clinical trials are necessary; generic drugs are not "identical" but sufficiently "similar". The similarities and differences of the drugs are questionable and quality of manufacturing of generics is a genuine concern.

"The proportion of branded vs. generic drug prescriptions dispensed in the U.S. has decreased since 2005. In 2005, some 40 percent of prescriptions dispensed were brand name drugs and around 50 percent of drugs dispensed were unbranded generic drugs. For comparison, in 2019, only some 10 percent of prescriptions were brand-name drugs while over 86 percent were unbranded generic drugs."[199]

We increasingly hear complaints of "they do not work as well" when switching from our usual brand drug to endless boxes of unfamiliar cheaper generic drugs, but perhaps the issue is one more complex and more dangerous than "they do not work as well." The problem lies in the number of different manufacturers making generic drugs and not specifically the fact they are generic. Each time we receive a generic, we might be receiving a different "make" of medication.

It is true that generic drugs must demonstrate bioequivalence to the brand-name original, however, two pills with the same amount of the same active therapeutic ingredient can cause different effects on the human body if they dissolve at different times in the stomach, if their active principles appear at different rates in the bloodstream, or if their excipients (binders, fillers, dyes and shellac coatings which are often of lower quality) influence the human body in different ways.

Generic medicines applications do not make use of any data from the originator (Brand drug) registration file. The data of originator products are never revealed to third parties so cannot be used by generic medicines researchers. Instead, generic medicines' producers research and develop their own formulation of the product. Regulators do not specifically regulate how quickly the medicine must reach maximum concentration in the blood, which is an important aspect of time-released medication that can impact its effectiveness. In short, the generic drug company only needs to test to prove it performs "similarly" to the brand drug. This needs to be done on only a few dozen healthy volunteers.

The interchangeability of some types of medication has been straight-forward but for some it has been complicated and contested. The British Generic Manufacturers Association (BGMA) is already warning about psychotropic generics and say "proceed with caution" with certain classes of drugs. They say making the switch with certain classes of drugs, and with drugs that have a narrow therapeutic range can pose potential problems and must be done with caution, if at all.

The FDA cites some psychotropic drugs for which generic formulations may not be interchangeable—including amitriptyline, perphenazine and venlafaxine—and others for which generic formulations may not be bioequivalent at all doses. It says the type of salt used to form a compound is also important and to avoid problems, physicians should prescribe generics containing the same salt as their brand-name counterpart!

In October 2009, the FDA declared that a generic drug it had previously approved, a generic version of the popular antidepressant Wellbutrin, was not in fact "bioequivalent" to the name-brand version. Complaints by patients the drug budeprion XL 300 mg. didn't work as effectively and made them feel sick had been dismissed for years by the FDA. However, an independent consumer laboratory tested the generic and found that it dumped the active ingredient into the bloodstream at four times the rate of the branded drug. The FDA took a highly unusual step, and it withdrew approval for the generic. It required other generic companies to retest their versions.

In 2008, a study "Did a switch to a generic antidepressant cause relapse?" was undertaken.[200] They concluded, "a switch to a generic form of an antidepressant, antipsychotic, mood stabilizer, or benzodiazepine, maintaining a concentration of only 80% of the original brand, might result in a sudden change in efficacy yielding an increased risk of withdrawal symptoms or even a relapse of a previously well-treated illness. Alternatively, if a patient is switched to a generic drug that maintains a 120% bioequivalence, there could be a sudden increase in adverse events. This could lead to a decrease in compliance and potentially prompt a clinician to misread the specific symptomatic presentation as a worsening of the symptoms. Considering such risks, it is disconcerting to note that patients and their physicians may not always realize that a switch has been made from a brand-name drug to a generic."

Anecdotal evidence tells us that changing generics made by different manufacturers can cause adverse effects. We know antidepressants "create" a chemical imbalance rather than "cure" one, but the question is, could the changes of generic drugs/different "makes" create new imbalances? Could some reports of nightmares, vomiting, anxiety, agitation, panic attacks, insomnia, irritability, hostility, impulsivity, akathisia, and mania in any way be linked to the quality and safety of generics? For some of us it seems certain generics can make us feel as if we have suddenly commenced an involuntary tapering of our medication. This is dangerous, as we know these drugs should not be stopped or reduced without the supervision of a medical professional. Failure to recognize switching between different makes of generics might cause symptoms similar to withdrawal is alarming.

Are generic antidepressants putting those of us dependent on medication at more risk of adverse effects? Are those of us attempting to withdraw from antidepressants particularly at risk? As an antidepressant's half-life is a crucial factor in managing withdrawal, do we need to be vigilant about prescribing different generics during tapering?

If generic antidepressants are "the same but not the same" as brand name antidepressants, it is time we understood the consequences of the strengths and limitations of the generic concept. We might choose a breakfast cereal with less fruit and plain packaging to save money, but it's not the same as having cheaper generic drugs chosen for us which might cause intolerance and psychological and physical adverse effects. More research and patient and prescriber awareness will enable us to determine under what circumstances is it safe to prescribe generics, substitute a brand name drug for a generic or switch manufacturers of generics. It is just one more issue to be added to the growing list of complexities associated with antidepressants, particularly withdrawal.

We should take a note of generic manufacturers' drugs we cannot tolerate and notify our prescriber. If we receive a generic/make which causes adverse effects we need to notify our prescriber or pharmacist immediately.

20
PRESCRIBING ANTIDEPRESSANTS TO CHILDREN AND YOUNG PEOPLE

Why are we medicating children with mind altering drugs? Is it time to question the morality of prescribing psychoactive antidepressants to children?

According to Dainius Pūras, "The tendency to medicalize children's distress can lead to an approach whereby multiple medications are prescribed for various symptoms, where some symptoms are iatrogenic effects of the medications, despite the lack of evidence for poly-pharmacy in children. Children have a right to thrive, to develop in a holistic way to their full potential and enjoy good physical and mental health in a sustainable world. It is crucial that investments are made to provide the nutritional, educational and societal resources for healthy development, and that the effects of adverse childhood experiences are addressed. It is important to train mental health professionals and educate broader society to understand that psychotropic medications are not effective first-choice treatment options in child and adolescent mental health care and that excessive use of psychotropic medications is not compliant with the right to health. A broad variety of other interventions, such as watchful waiting and other psychosocial interventions, must be available, accessible, acceptable and of sufficient quality."[201]

We know that there is rarely any biological justification for prescribing antidepressants to anyone of any age. We know these drugs create a chemical imbalance rather than cure one. We know the effects of these drugs can be severe and long lasting and can increase suicidality. We know the mental health diagnoses given to children are labels created by psychiatry. So why does the medicalizing of child behavior and emotions continue to be booming business for the pharmaceutical industry, with millions of children and young adults being prescribed antidepressants in the US and developed nations?

The pharmaceutical industry views young people as an antidepressant mass market. Parents and care providers who make decisions on their behalf have generally already bought into the pharmaceutical sales pitch of our sadness, anxiety or loneliness being medical issues.

Cultural behavior puts parents in a "damned if you do and damned if you don't" dilemma, with our children's health and wellbeing at stake.

In 2003, the UK Medicine and Healthcare Regulatory Agency (MHRA) decided it would only recommend fluoxetine for patients under 18 because of unfavorable risk benefit profiles for all other SSRI antidepressants.[202] Following this, in 2004, the FDA announced, "Today the Food and Drug Administration (FDA) directed manufacturers of all antidepressant drugs to revise the labeling for their products to include a boxed warning and expanded warning statements that alert health care providers to an increased risk of suicidality (suicidal thinking and behavior) in children and adolescents being treated with these agents, and to include additional information about the results of pediatric studies."[203]

A Boxed Warning or Black Box warning is the FDA Warning on a drug Patient Information Leaflet indicating the drug has a serious risk of adverse effect which can be life-threatening. But even with their Black Box Warning, the FDA continue to say, "Don't leave childhood depression untreated." They view depression as an illness with associated behaviors. They have a somewhat confusing message focusing on their belief they are treating an "illness", even though we know there are no tests of any kind to prove depression is biological.

"Some parents might think that medication is the solution for depression-related problem behavior. In fact, that's not the case. The Food and Drug Administration hasn't approved any drugs solely for the treatment of "behavior problems." When the FDA approves a drug for depression—whether for adults or children—it's to treat the illness, not the behavior associated with it. There are multiple parts to mental illness, and the symptoms are usually what drug companies study and what parents worry about. But it's rare for us at FDA to target just one part of the illness," says Mitchell Mathis, M.D., a psychiatrist who is the Director of FDA's Division of Psychiatry Products.[204]

The following is the type of general information we might see online regarding children and antidepressant prescribing, telling us antidepressants don't even need to be FDA approved for our children. "There are two antidepressants that the FDA has approved for use in children or teens to treat depression: Prozac (fluoxetine) for kids 8 and older and Lexapro (escitalopram) for kids 12 and older. Additionally, Zoloft (sertraline), Luvox (fluvoxamine), and Anafranil (clomipramine) have been approved along with Prozac to treat kids with obsessive-compulsive disorder (OCD). Just because a medication is not FDA-approved doesn't mean that your doctor won't prescribe it, particularly if you have an older child. Physicians often prescribe other antidepressants for children and teens that are not FDA-approved because they have been proven to be effective and fairly safe. Be sure to read the medication guide that comes with your child's antidepressant to find out more information, such as risks, side effects, and cautions."[205]

Not only are we misinformed about the potential dangers of prescribing antidepressants to our children, but we are encouraged to look out for and have our children screened for signs of mental illness, all pointing to whether or not a child might need a "medical professional". These are promoted as simple tests or "General Mental Health Screening Tools", but they might see our children on the life-changing road to becoming lifelong psychiatric patients.

"Screening tools such as these can help you begin to make sense of what your child is experiencing. Remember, these assessments are not an official diagnosis but rather a guide for helping you discern whether or not your child may benefit from a formal evaluation or consultation with a medical professional. If you or your child complete any of these assessments, bring them with you to your appointment with a medical or mental health professional as they will find the information very helpful. These screening tools can be an important step in your family getting the support it needs and the professional treatment your child needs."[206]

Despite the often laid-back attitude towards children and antidepressants, "fairly safe" being commonly used, data concerning the safety and efficacy of antidepressant use for children is far from reassuring. There have been disturbing reports of SSRI trials and young people, alleging drug companies hid unfavorable data, exaggerated the benefits and hid the adverse effects, in particular the risk of suicidality.

In the short-term clinical trials of SSRIs, 4% of the medicated youth became suicidal, which was double the rate for those on placebo. This led the FDA to put a black box warning on antidepressants that they increased the risk of a suicidal event. In a large NIMH study, known as the TADs study, 22% of adolescents treated with an SSRI had a suicide event, compared with 6.7% of those not taking the drug. Seventeen of the 18 youths who attempted suicide during the study were taking an antidepressant.[207]

Research in Australia has revealed an alarming link between rising antidepressant use and suicide rates among young Australians; "the research examined Australian antidepressant prescribing and suicide rates since controversial warnings by the US Food and Drug Administration (FDA), in 2004 and 2007, that the use of antidepressants by people under 25 years of age with depression was associated with approximately double the risk of suicidal thoughts and behaviors."[208]

There is particular concern over the increase in prescribing to children during Covid-19. "One option is watchful waiting, where parents and doctors closely monitor the young person and avoid exposing them to the extra risk of suicidality identified by the FDA and TGA. Throwing petrol on an already out of control fire is rarely a good idea. Nonetheless, between July 2017 and June 2018, over 100,000 (1.8%) Australians under 18 were prescribed an antidepressant. Some received these drugs for anxiety, but many were prescribed them off-label for depression."[209]

AntiDepAware is a website posting articles and links to reports of inquests of more than 5500 self-inflicted deaths related to the use of antidepressants. These are the tip of the iceberg of actual cases worldwide.

The site says many of the people who died by suicide had not been depressed but had been prescribed antidepressants for conditions such as anxiety, insomnia, PTSD, work-based stress or grief. It is important we note the very large number of children and young people who are featured on this site and their deaths linked to the antidepressants they had been prescribed.

There is a very real chance that children prescribed antidepressants will possibly experience mood instability sufficient to attract a label of bipolar disorder. A 2004 study at Yale University, found the risk was particularly pronounced for children and adolescents.

The use of an antidepressant increased the conversion risk seven-fold for children 5 to 9 years old, four-fold for those 10 to 14 years old, and slightly more than two-fold for those 15 to 19 years old.[210] The apparent rise in prevalence of "bipolar" in young adults in the US is very concerning.

Some things just don't make sense. In an age where we obsess over food additives, protecting our children on-line, keeping them safe from bullies and plastering them from head to toe in sunscreen, why do we pay so little attention to the growing trend of prescribing mind-altering antidepressants to children and young people? Why are we allowing children to believe they are mentally ill and their problems can be solved by popping psychoactive pills?

As parents we need education. None of us wish to harm our children, but we are brainwashed by societal beliefs and the medical profession in whom we put our trust. Instead of seeing our children as needing medication, we need to help our children deal with suffering as part of life, part of growing up. Whilst psychiatry says ordinary distress and sadness is mental illness, we must teach children that however painful their distress may be, it is, more often than not their normal reactions to the difficulties of everyday life. Nothing is more cruel than allowing children to believe they are mentally ill and their problems can be solved by antidepressants.

Children are very rarely genuinely mentally ill. More often they are subjected to social causes of anxiety or sadness. General feelings of helplessness because of poverty, family and peer relationships, loneliness, pressure from school and social media are the norm in today's society and yet we continuing to treat children as if they have psychiatric disorders.

Prescribing antidepressants to children is incompatible with "Building Resilient Kids", a mantra heard throughout education and social care. Telling children they can be resilient when faced with poverty, broken and dysfunctional families and overwhelming societal and educational pressures is one tool used by governments and the powers that be. Antidepressants are just one more. Things go wrong when children don't live up to the expectations of today's society. It seems it is sometimes simply easier for some parents to buy into the false dangerous narrative that, just like adults, children have a chemical imbalance causing depression. Shouldn't we be questioning why it all points to the child or their brain being at fault and it is the child, not society which needs to be cured?

The United Nations Convention on the Rights of the Child (UNCRC) sets out the fundamental rights of all children and young people. "Nearly 25 years ago, the world made a promise to children: that we would do everything in our power to protect and promote their rights to survive and thrive, to learn and grow, to make their voices heard and to reach their full potential. The Convention changed the way children are viewed and treated—i.e., as human beings with a distinct set of rights instead of as passive objects of care and charity." Ironically, Article 33 of the UNCRC states, "You have the right to be protected from dangerous drugs."

By encouraging children to believe they are broken and are to blame for their distress and by medicating them with powerful drugs we know change brain chemistry, are we taking away their right to survive, and ability to thrive, be protected and reach their full potential? At what point in their life might a child question their medication? When they do, what damage might already have been done? Parents have a responsibility to learn the truth about antidepressants and their unknown effects on a developing brain. Does any parent have the right to control the development of their child with drugs? The reality is that children parked on antidepressants at a young age become medicated adults. At some point they will make up their own mind about their medication, might find themselves battling prescribed drug dependence or they simply might not like the way they turned out.

Meanwhile, back at the FDA, "Kids just don't have time to leave their depression untreated. The social and educational consequences of a lengthy recovery are huge. They could fail a grade. They could lose all of their friends." (Child and adolescent psychiatrist Tiffany R. Farchione, M.D., is the Acting Deputy Director of FDA's Division of Psychiatry Products.)

By now, reading this book, we understand the real potential health and social consequences of choosing to treat our children with antidepressants. They could lose so much more than "all of their friends."

WARNING: "Pediatric patients being treated with antidepressants for any indication should be closely observed for clinical worsening, as well as agitation, irritability, suicidality, and unusual changes in behavior, especially during the initial few months of a course of drug therapy, or at times of dose changes, either increases or decreases. This monitoring should include daily observation by families and caregivers and frequent contact with the physician. It is also recommended that prescriptions for antidepressants be written for the smallest quantity of tablets consistent with good patient management, in order to reduce the risk of overdose."[211]

21
THE ELDERLY, VULNERABILITY AND ANTIDEPRESSANTS

Our elderly are vulnerable victims of the system. At a time when they deserve care and social support, why are we choosing psychoactive medication over human interaction and kindness?

"Treatment of mental disorders among older Americans has become a major public health need. The number of people over the age of 65 with psychiatric disorders will more than double by the year 2030, from 7 million in 2000 to 15 million. The past decade has seen dramatic growth in research on the causes and treatments of the psychiatric problems of older adults."[212]

Our senior citizens are perhaps the most vulnerable when it comes to being diagnosed mentally ill. It seems quite obvious that older people are those most likely to suffer from loneliness, isolation, sadness, anxiety and the range of feelings which accompany elderly life and the many changes it presents. Many suffer from insecurity, from stigma and abuse, ageism, sexism and lack of confidence due to the physical and cognitive difficulties which come naturally with old age.

Published in the Journal of the American Geriatrics Society, geriatric mental health leaders wrote, "COVID-19 Pandemic and Ageism: A Call for Humanitarian Care."[213] But don't our elderly deserve humanitarian care at all times? Today's society can sometimes be difficult to tolerate and navigate for most of us, but instead of providing the elderly with said "humanitarian care", why do we choose to treat our elderly population with antidepressants and other psychiatric drugs?

In 2011, a study published in the British Medical Journal raised questions about antidepressant risks and the over 65s. Its conclusions were that taking antidepressants was associated with increased death rates and other adverse consequences, and that the new antidepressants may have greater serious risks than those associated with previous generations of antidepressants. They determined SSRI and related antidepressants "were associated with an increased risk of several adverse outcomes compared with tricyclic antidepressants".

"The average age of participants was 75. Many suffered from other illness, including heart disease and diabetes, and were taking multiple medications. Nearly 90 percent of patients were prescribed an antidepressant during the study period. Of those, 55 percent received SSRIs, 32 percent received TCAs, and 13.5 percent received other antidepressants. Those taking SSRIs had an increased risk of stroke, falls, fracture, epilepsy or seizures, high levels of salt in the blood and dying of any cause, compared with those taking TCAs."[214]

A UK study in the British Journal of Psychiatry reported new antidepressant prescribing to over 65s has doubled over twenty years. This was, despite the fact that the number of people diagnosed with depression in this age group had changed very little. Professor Anthony Arthur of the university of East Anglia said "Substantial increases in prescribing have not reduced the prevalence of depression in the over-65 population. The causes of depression in older people, the factors that perpetuate it, and the best ways to manage it remain poorly understood and merit more attention."[215]

Older people taking antidepressants are at more risk of dying or suffering strokes, falls, fractures and epilepsy, as well as the many other adverse effects commonly suffered in other age groups. Elderly with heart conditions, diabetes, previous strokes and other conditions have antidepressants prescribed on top of other medications putting them at risk of serious adverse drug interactions.

The American Academy of Neurology study, "Association of anticholinergic medications and AD biomarkers with incidence of MCI among cognitively normal older adults," highlighted the adverse impact of anticholinergic medications on cognition and the need for deprescribing trials, particularly among individuals with elevated risk for Alzheimer's Disease.[216]

There are so many reasons why it does not make sense to medicate our elderly with drugs which are not fit for purpose. Despite the fact they are generally more sensitive to drugs, our aging population is an easy target for overprescribing. It has been reported prescribing to the elderly in care homes and assisted living has increased fourfold with around double the number of women treated with an antidepressant compared to men; (24.3 percent of all women aged 60 and above). The many serious potential adverse effects alone which can include, Cognitive Brain Impairment, dementia, diabetes, tardive dysphoria and worsening of depression, should make us question prescribing to aging individuals with existing health conditions.

Millions of us will take our antidepressant dependence with us into old age. Education is once again key to supporting us throughout our medication journey. As we become older, we might be dependent on antidepressants we have taken for many years. A change in circumstances might put us in a position where we are no longer able to manage our unrecognized dependence. Care providers might lack knowledge of the dangers of antidepressant dependence. We might become vulnerable to being harmed by changes to or withdrawal of medication; it might be increased or withdrawn at any time, without informed consent. Just as with people in other age groups, our elderly, when first prescribed, probably do not have a chemical imbalance causing their depression. What they do generally have is difficulty coping with life and the changes it presents with growing old. For many, the reality of their condition might be as simple as one of loneliness.

MDLinx, reports "The newest epidemic in America now affects up to 47% of adults—double the number affected a few decades ago."[217] Loneliness is not a mental illness but is certainly being treated that way as we continue to overmedicate our elderly. It is just one more example of today's medicalization of a natural but totally avoidable state we need to prevent rather than "treat". "Psychologists, psychiatrists, and social scientists have known from clinical work over decades that both intellectual and social engagement help to prevent loneliness."[218] We also know social activity is positively associated with a decrease in cognitive decline.

Drugs are a cheap and easy option compared to talking therapies. Talking therapies are very often unavailable, have long waiting lists or are expensive and doctors rarely refer older people for therapy. The fact is there is a severe lack of provision of psychosocial services and interventions for the elderly which is perhaps fueled by our reliance on antidepressants. There is once again a huge need for a change in practice when it comes to treating our senior citizens. Treating our ability to cope with life and calling it mental illness as we get older is both disrespectful and counterproductive. We need a societal change. Whilst medication can help some older people, is it time for organizations such as the National Institute on Aging to rethink their adoption of the "medical model of mental health" approach? Is it time we look first at the individual and not at their so called real "illness", "clinical" depression, "disorder", or whichever label fits to make the system easier?

To quote the National Institute of Aging, "When you have depression, you have trouble with daily life for weeks at a time. Doctors call this condition "depressive disorder" or "clinical depression". "Depression is a real illness. It is not a sign of a person's weakness or a character flaw. You can't 'snap out of' clinical depression. Most people who experience depression need treatment to get better."[219] This is a just one more example of the damaging, societally accepted narrative we need to change.

22

ANTIDEPRESSANTS, THE ARMED FORCES, PTSD AND SUICIDE

The Armed Forces, PTSD, antidepressants and suicide: don't those who serve us deserve better?

Around 8 million adults are diagnosed with Post-Traumatic Stress Disorder (PTSD) during a given year. Perhaps the most tragic consequences of PTSD are felt by our military.

Throughout history soldiers have inevitably returned from wars with traumatic memories but until the emergence of PTSD, they would generally use their personal resilience, community support and the passing of time to rebuild their lives. PTSD turned military experience and human suffering into a disease; a disease needing drugs. In what is a pitiful commercial venture, the pharmaceutical industry and psychiatry see the military as their target, they take aim and boom... another successful psychiatric drug market is created and developed. It was one more area of human suffering ripe for exploitation and medicalization.

The use of psychological interventions is recommended as a first-line approach for PTSD by a range of authoritative sources but, in reality, our veterans are usually medicated when returning from active duty.[221] There are four antidepressants recommended for PTSD: sertraline (Zoloft), paroxetine (Paxil), fluoxetine (Prozac), and venlafaxine (Effexor).

In addition to an initial diagnosis, the US Department of Veteran Affairs (VA), states; "Most people with PTSD—about 80%—have one or more additional mental health diagnoses. They are also at risk for functional impairments, reduced quality of life, and relationship problems. PTSD and trauma are linked to physical health problems as well. These articles explain the connections among PTSD, trauma and co-occurring mental and physical health problems."[222] Knowing what we do about the adverse effects of antidepressants and the prescribing cascade they can cause; is it any surprise veterans are at risk of so many other impairments and health problems?

Primary Care PTSD Screen for DSM-5 (PC-PTSD-5)[224]

Description

The Primary Care PTSD Screen for DSM-5 (PC-PTSD-5) is a 5-item screen that was designed for use in primary care settings. The measure begins with an item designed to assess whether the respondent has had any exposure to traumatic events. If a respondent denies exposure, the PC-PTSD-5 is complete with a score of 0. However, if a respondent indicates that they have experienced a traumatic event over the course of their life, the respondent is instructed to respond to five additional yes/no questions about how that trauma exposure has affected them over the past month.

Scale

Sometimes things happen to people that are unusually or especially frightening, horrible, or traumatic. For example:

- A serious accident or fire
- A physical or sexual assault or abuse
- An earthquake or flood
- A war
- Seeing someone be killed or seriously injured
- Having a loved one die through homicide or suicide

Have you ever experienced this kind of event? YES / NO
If no, screen total = 0. Please stop here.
If yes, please answer the questions below.

In the past month, have you...

- Had nightmares about the event(s) or thought about the event(s) when you didnot want to? YES / NO

- Tried hard not to think about the event(s) or went out of your way to avoid situations that reminded you of the event(s)? YES / NO
- Been constantly on guard, watchful, or easily startled? YES / NO
- Felt numb or detached from people, activities, or your surroundings? YES / NO
- Felt guilty or unable to stop blaming yourself or others for the event(s) or any problems the event(s) may have caused? YES / NO

Miriam Reisman writes, "Complicating the diagnosis and assessment of PTSD in military veterans are the high rates of psychiatric comorbidity. Depression is the most common comorbidity of PTSD in veterans. Results from a large national survey show that major depressive disorder (MDD) is nearly three to five times more likely to emerge in those with PTSD than those without PTSD. A large meta-analysis composed of 57 studies, across both military and civilian samples, found an MDD and PTSD comorbidity rate of 52%."[223]

The National Center for PTSD provides a number of "PTSD Screening Instruments" (brief questionnaires), to help identify people who are more likely to have PTSD. These simplistic tools, created with the DSM-5, are very similar to the tools used to screen for other disorders in the general population. Their primary aim is to diagnose a condition which needs medication.

Alarmingly, instead of questioning the current overprescribing, we are seeing more clinical trials to develop and approve other drugs to treat PTSD. It has become a very lucrative arm of the pharmaceutical industry's psychiatric drug market. PTSD is easy to understand and relate to by anyone who has suffered trauma or an adverse life event and using it, our military and veterans are particularly at risk of being medicated, often with serious or fatal consequences.

There have been more than 70,000 veteran suicides since 2006 and given it is widely acknowledged that prescription drugs can put us at risk of dangerous adverse effects, most notably that antidepressants and some other medication can raise the risk of suicide, should we be questioning the connection between the high rates of prescribing to veterans and number of veterans ending their lives by suicide?

Robert Whitaker and Derek Blumke published a report detailing VA suicide data which shows an increased risk of suicide for veterans treated at the VA.[225] It also highlights disproportionately high rates of prescribing to veterans of psychiatric drugs which we know increase suicide risk. Despite the VA declaring "preventing suicide among Veterans is the VA's top clinical priority", Whitaker and Blumke write, "Its screening protocols have ushered an ever greater number of veterans into psychiatric care, where treatment with antidepressants and other psychiatric drugs is regularly prescribed. Suicide rates have increased in lockstep with the increased exposure among veterans to such medications." This of course is the exact same message given to the general public; that suicide is a public health issue, we need to identify mental health problems, diagnose them and treat them.

In 2016, the VA published a report they said was the "most comprehensive analysis of Veteran suicide in our nation's history." They divided VHA-using patients into four subgroups: Undiagnosed and Untreated (for a mental health or substance abuse disorder), Undiagnosed and Treated (with either a psychiatric drug or non-pharmacologic treatment), Diagnosed and Untreated, and Diagnosed and Treated.

The results show those without a diagnosis who got mental health treatment were more likely to die by suicide than those without a diagnosis who did not access such treatment. In 2014, those who got treatment died at twice the rate of the "untreated" group. Most concerningly, those who had no diagnosis but received mental health treatment were more likely to die by suicide than those with an untreated diagnosis. The findings show exactly why mental health treatment is doubling the risk of suicide, something we already know from clinical trials.

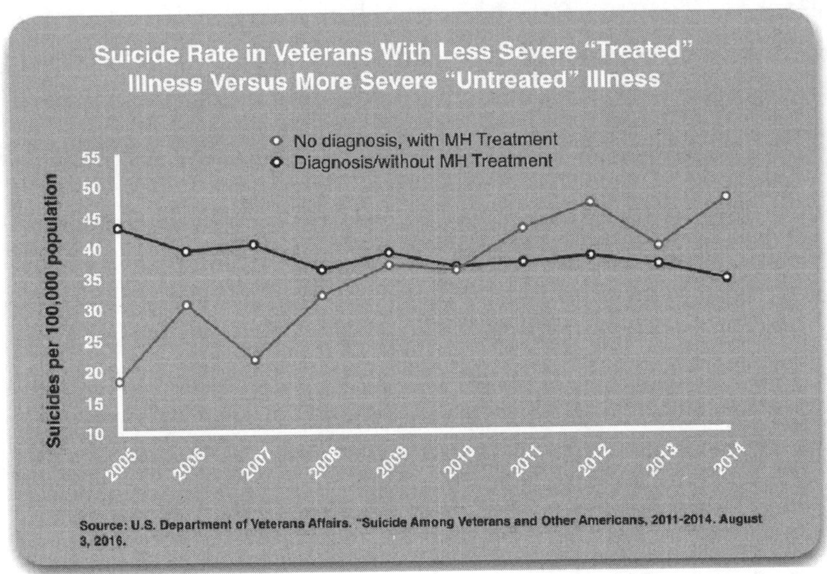

Source: U.S. Department of Veterans Affairs. "Suicide Among Veterans and Other Americans, 2011-2014. August 3, 2016.

More than 53,000 veterans died by gun suicide between 2005 and 2016 and Americans are quick to point the finger at the accessibility of guns.[226] But there are a multitude of factors contributing to suicide. Many are quick to blame the access to guns as a cause of the high rates of suicide in the US, but few are prepared to acknowledge the overprescribing of prescription drugs as a key factor.

"It's a daunting list," Dr. Sue Sisley, a psychiatrist in Phoenix, told The Huffington Post about the staggering number of medications available for PTSD. The Department of Veterans Affairs' national formulary is a catalog of drugs and supplies commonly prescribed by VA doctors overall and it contains more than 1,500 items. "When I show this list to our military veterans, they were completely nauseated because they have frequently been the target of so many of these medication trials, Many of the medications used to treat serious PTSD symptoms such as anxiety, depression, flashbacks and insomnia come with risky side effects, especially when combined with one another. One of the most dangerous is an increase in suicidal thinking."[227]

But are things changing and are questions starting to be asked about prescription drugs and veterans' mental health treatment? Mad in America has launched the Veterans, Service Members & Military Families Initiative, to help the community become better educated and to assist service members, veterans and their families to identify alternatives to the dominant drug-based model of mental health. The Veterans of Foreign Wars (VFW) and the American Legion are also looking at antidepressants and the suicides of service members, veterans and their families.[228]

A new approach, Warfighter Advance, founded by Dr. Mary Neal Vieten is leading the way in offering an alternative way to help veterans. Its aim is "100% successful reintegration & resilience of the Warfighter and a world where a traumatized Warfighter is fully restored in a non-medical context."[229] It openly rejects the medical model of treating trauma with medication and recognizes the need for informed consent to mental health care. It offers tools to help with post-deployment life empowering military personnel (active or veteran), to help build support, relationships and the confidence to live meaningful lives.

"After a careful analysis of the risk-benefit ratio, we reject all 'mental illness' labels for the Warfighter and, likewise, reject the use or usefulness of psychiatric medications in the process of Warfighter reintegration. We acknowledge the devastating implications of these labels and 'treatments' for traumatized individuals in general."

"Warfighter Advance changes the trajectory of the warfighter's post-deployment life, so that rather than an existence characterized by an endless cycle of mental illness diagnoses, medications, medical appointments and disappointments, the warfighter has a life characterized by pride, productivity, healthy relationships, continued service, and advocacy for the same outcomes for their fellow service members."

The 20 veterans who die every day by suicide in the US are clear evidence of the urgent need for change. Veterans deserve our current societal approach to "suicide prevention" to be questioned and we need to acknowledge screening, diagnosis and treating with antidepressants are often a precursor to suicide.

It is time to change the predominant messages such as those of "The American Foundation for Suicide Prevention" who openly tell us "ninety percent of people who die by suicide have a mental disorder at the time of their deaths." Instead of questioning how many are taking mind altering psychoactive antidepressants with a black box warning for suicidal ideation, they continue to promote medical diagnoses and treatment as a way to reduce suicide. They continue to propagate the message that medication is best. "The most common disorder associated with suicide, the Foundation states "is depression, an illness that goes undiagnosed and untreated far too often." It advises the media to "convey that suicidal thoughts and behaviors can be reduced with the proper mental health support and treatment."[230]

What would happen if we were to see a massive reduction in the mental health messages we constantly hear, reductions in the diagnosis of the disorders accompanying them and reductions in the prescribing of the harmful antidepressants some of us unnecessarily swallow? What would happen if we all became "Warfighters" and took a different approach to changing and adapting to the challenges in our lives? Paradoxically speaking, the more drugs prescribed the more suicides there will be... but we might not hear this message from government bodies or the medical profession any time soon.

PART 5

Patient Experiences

PATIENT EXPERIENCES

> "Next time you see a TV commercial for a prescription drug, remind yourself that you know nothing about medical treatment and that everybody who made the commercial has a financial interest in your future behavior."[231]

THE PHARMACEUTICAL INDUSTRY is one of the biggest advertising spenders in the United States. (The US and New Zealand are the only two developed world countries to allow pharmaceutical direct to consumer advertising (DTCA) on TV.) In 2017, in the New York Times, Joanna Kaufman asked us, "Think You're Seeing More Drug Ads on TV? You Are, and Here's Why."[232] In 2018, Jacob Bell wrote, "Just considering television, 187 commercials for about 70 prescription medications have collectively aired almost half a million times since the start of 2018. And to do that, drug companies shelled out $2.8 billion, according to marketing analytics provider iSpot.tv."[233]

November 2015, the American Medical Association (AMA) called for a ban on direct-to-consumer advertising of prescription drugs and medical devices, including television advertisements. Their main justification was they "encourage patients to ask for costlier drugs that may not be appropriate for them"![234] "A new STAT-Harvard poll indicates that the AMA's position has clear majority support from the American public. According to the poll, 57 percent of Americans favored removing pharma ads from TV; 39 percent were opposed. 44 percent of those polled also said the FDA should be allowed not to approve a new drug if it considers the price too high."[235]

The drug commercials usually tell a specific type of personal story. The character is of course an attractive if supposedly ailing individual with a smile to die for. They are being saved by the drug which is enabling them to live perfectly in their ideal suburban world. None of this is real, of course. Actor patients with fake illness seeing actor doctors with the air of George Clooney. It's all polished, idealistic and any "side effects" are delivered in rapid fire, accompanied by text requiring binoculars. We have no idea which "side effects" are the most dangerous, the severity of them or the frequency of them.

As the editors of Scientific American tell us, "Peddling pharmaceuticals on TV is a lousy form of health education, and it can also drive up medical costs."[236] It is, without doubt, the most irresponsible way to educate consumers about medication, in particular antidepressants and other "psychiatric drugs", portraying the wonderful life we can all have if we just swallow that pill. All our stresses, anxiety and sadness will disappear when we buy into the idea of having shiny hair, a perfect apartment and an adoring partner. As the commercials entice us, the need to actually understand and learn about the medication before we take it seems irrelevant. The unrealistically simple yet persuasive messaging is all it takes for us to visit our doctor with the name of that medication firmly planted in our mind.

The pharmaceutical industry wants us to believe their commercials empower, educate and ensure we have confidence in their products, when in reality they are selling us drugs we can often do without. Their advertising is one of the most effective drivers in the medicalization of the United States and works with screening and diagnosing as part of their billion-dollar marketing toolbox.

The juxtaposition of the actor patient and the real-life patient is frightening. We are sold a quick fix and a miracle cure when in reality, we often consent to a medicated life of adverse effects, prolonged and additional illness and sometimes death. We know it is impossible to predict how we will react to antidepressants and nowhere in any antidepressant commercial are we told this. Some of us might find them useful, if taken for the shortest time but many of us will find the drugs we buy into do significantly more harm than good. Eventually we will need the information we should have received before we agreed (without informed consent) to take them. It is usually only when things go wrong that we seek more information, and we look for help and support.

Anecdotal evidence is the best evidence we have when it comes to learning about the sometimes devastating effects of antidepressants. The personal experiences of people worldwide who have experienced a life "antidepressed"[237] tell a very different story to the ones we are sold in the TV commercials. These are real people who believed what they were told by the medical profession, took antidepressants as prescribed and whose lives will never be the same again. Such experiences were looked at in the research study, "The Patient Voice", published in Therapeutic Advances in Psychopharmacology.[238]

Amongst their findings, "A total of 97% of respondents were offered a prescription on their initial consultation with a doctor, 5% reported being offered talking therapy, and 0.6% were offered lifestyle advice (with some patients offered more than one option)."

"When patients reported side effects to their physician, the response of their doctor varied widely: 32% tried an alternative drug, 35% added another drug, 28% adjusted the dosage, and in 21% of cases the doctor dismissed the idea that the side effects were related to the prescribed drug."

"The researchers found the following common themes:[239]

A lack of information given to patients about the risk of antidepressant withdrawal.

Doctors failing to recognize the symptoms of withdrawal.

Doctors being poorly informed about the best method of tapering prescribed medications. Patients being diagnosed with a relapse of the underlying condition or medical illnesses other than withdrawal.

Patients seeking advice outside of mainstream healthcare, including from online forums.

Significant effects on functioning for those experiencing withdrawal."

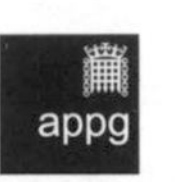

PATIENT EXPERIENCES OF PRESCRIBED DRUG DEPENDENCE –

Patient Journey Map: Initial Prescription and Outcomes

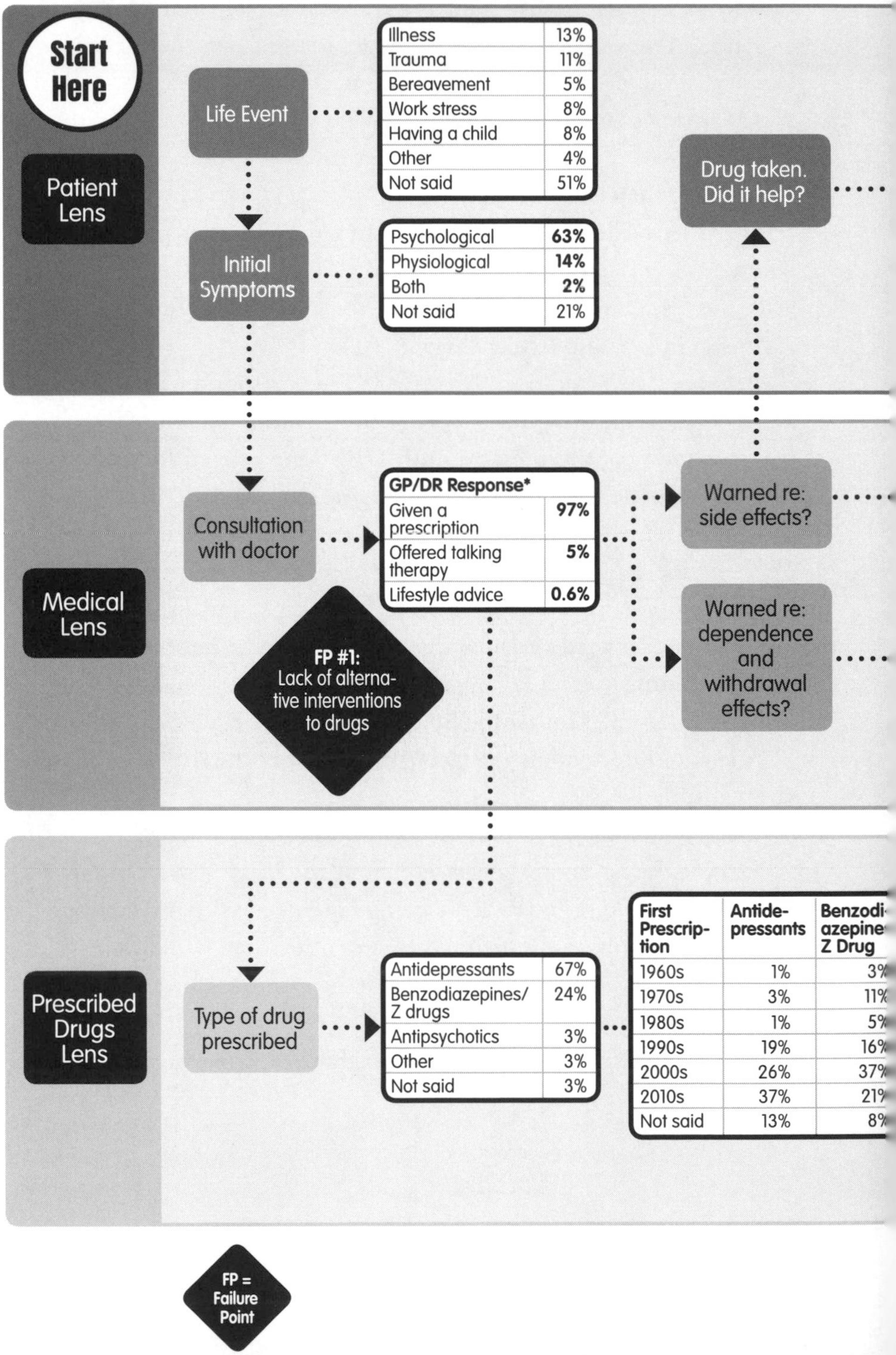

Start Here

Patient Lens

Life Event

Illness	13%
Trauma	11%
Bereavement	5%
Work stress	8%
Having a child	8%
Other	4%
Not said	51%

Initial Symptoms

Psychological	**63%**
Physiological	**14%**
Both	**2%**
Not said	21%

Drug taken. Did it help?

Medical Lens

Consultation with doctor

GP/DR Response*	
Given a prescription	**97%**
Offered talking therapy	**5%**
Lifestyle advice	**0.6%**

FP #1: Lack of alternative interventions to drugs

Warned re: side effects?

Warned re: dependence and withdrawal effects?

Prescribed Drugs Lens

Type of drug prescribed

Antidepressants	67%
Benzodiazepines/ Z drugs	24%
Antipsychotics	3%
Other	3%
Not said	3%

First Prescription	Antidepressants	Benzodiazepine Z Drug
1960s	1%	3%
1970s	3%	11%
1980s	1%	5%
1990s	19%	16%
2000s	26%	37%
2010s	37%	21%
Not said	13%	8%

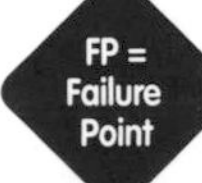

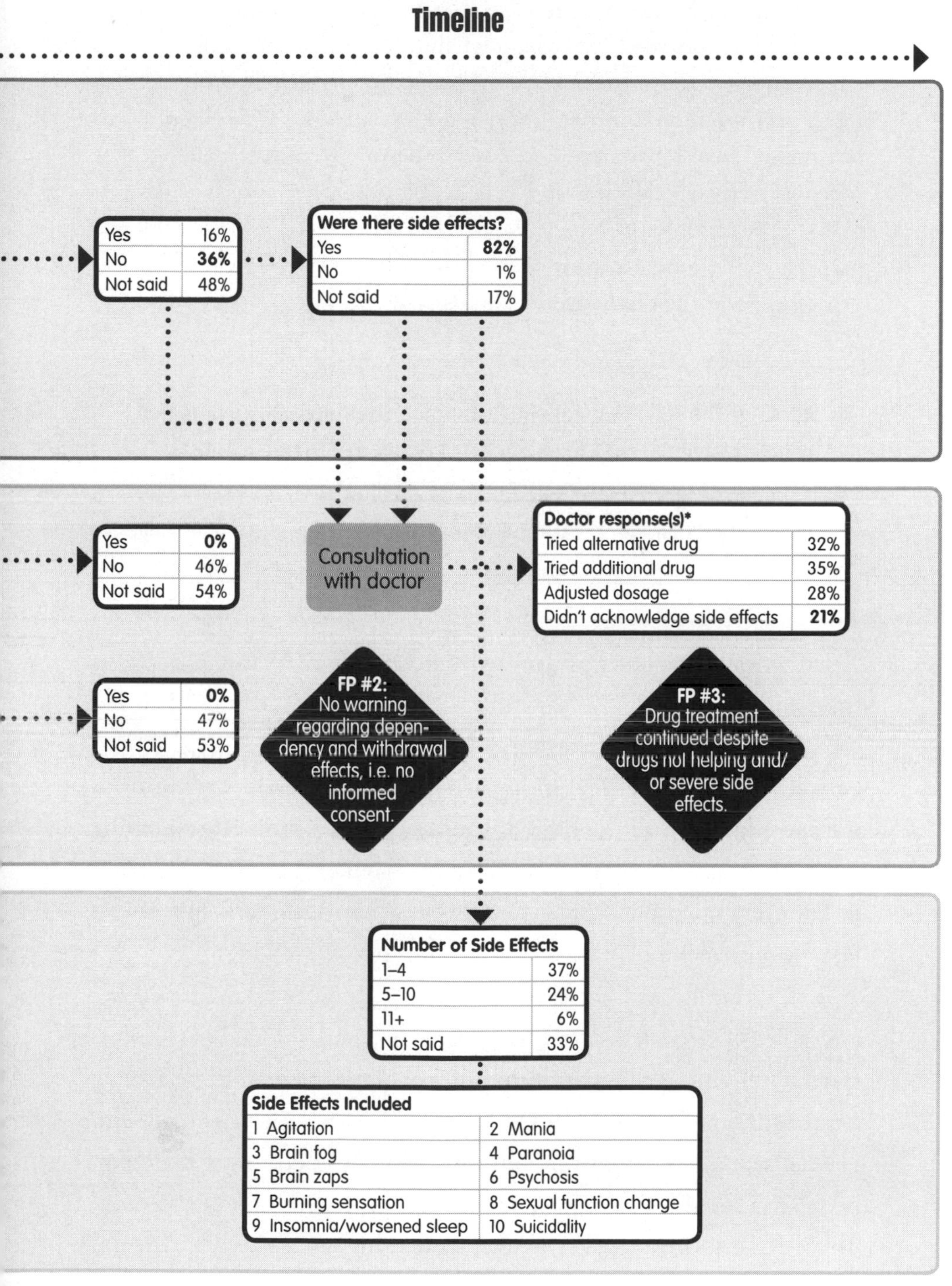

* Up to three answers recorded per petition responder. Percentage is equal to percent of 158 responders who mentioned each answer.

The study shows the failure of the medical profession to listen to patients. It shows their lack of knowledge about antidepressant adverse effects and withdrawal. These are the professionals we rely on to help us make decisions about our healthcare and it is obvious, when it comes to our mental health, we need and deserve better. We must challenge our preconceived societal ideas and beliefs about antidepressants and learn from the experiences of others. We need to understand real-life evidence paints a very different picture to the one often portrayed by the medical profession and the pharmaceutical industry.

Warning: The following patient testimonials feature sensitive topics, including suicide, substance-related trauma and emotional distress. This content may be upsetting for some readers and may exacerbate underlying symptoms. Please use your best judgment when proceeding.

"I am writing this letter, so you will understand the harm and deaths from antidepressants. On September 8, 2011, my 42 year old beloved son took his life. I couldn't wrap my mind around how this could even be true. He wasn't suicidal in his life. He lived across the street from me and I saw him all the time, I would know as a mom, if something was bothering him. As you can probably imagine, I asked my daughter in-law every question I could think of, to get a reason to WHY. If you lose a family member to suicide, you want to know WHY!

Everything I asked her, she said no to. Finally, one day I called her and asked if he was taking any medications and she said yes, Zoloft (sertraline) and Wellbutrin (bupropion). I asked her, was he feeling depressed? She told me in 1999 he saw his PA and was diagnosed with generalized anxiety; that through the years, he tried to get off them, because of the side effects he suffered with, only to not be able to do it. Then, in the spring of 2011, he told his wife he wanted his life back and called his doctor to get tapered off them. I have had to learn the hard way that doctors taper their patients too fast. I'm sure you have heard this from most of the people who have written to you.

A few months later withdrawals hit him, which is typical with antidepressants. More anxiety and not being able to sleep. This probably caused him to feel depressed, and so he called his doctor to go back on them, not knowing it was the antidepressants that caused his problems. NINE DAYS AFTER RESTARTING ZOLOFT (SERTRALINE) HE SHOT HIMSELF! I would love to tell you about his day before he suddenly and so out of character ended his life, leaving a widow and two children fatherless. Something needs to be done, as too many people have taken their lives or other lives."

—From Petition Ref LLLLLLL

"Everyone has some emotional problems, of varying degrees. I sure had my fair share since I can remember, all had a root cause, all had a reason. But I did not know how to deal with them, no one was able to guide me, to comfort me, teach me proper coping skills. I thought, I am different, something is wrong with me. Lousy childhood, abandoned by father, further inept parenting, lousy husband, the confusing life-circle continued. What was wrong with me? Because I cried too much, asked too many questions, received stoned silence, insomnia, fearful of dark shadows that crept in the night which sometimes were really not shadows at all. I tried to verbalize these feelings, fears, anxieties, challenges, because I wanted to connect, talking and having someone to listen, to believe, even parents, even husband, even doctors, put up barriers, they did not want to hear, nor did they know what to say. "Let's just shove some pills down your throat."

Mother said, "You are the crazy one, you are seeing a psychiatrist, nothing wrong with me, it is something wrong with you." I shut myself off, feeling ostracized, feeling like a bad person. So thus it went on, post-partum antidepressants that just made me so drowsy, I could not care for my young baby, unresolved marital situation that ended in divorce. If I could only talk, if only someone would listen, if only someone would validate me and my feelings, if only I was told, that it was all part and parcel of living, instead of being "tranquilized", mouth was so dry, head foggy, wobbly legs, I could not speak, if I could. I walked around in a daze, barely participating.

Later on there was Prozac, a touted miracle drug (got bad press because caused some suicidal deaths) and that was ignored, and then after ten years, Cymbalta, supposedly another miracle drug for its wonderful chronic pain alleviation. And then came my decision to withdraw from Cymbalta after being on it for 8 years. Nightmares, physical feelings of one leg draining into the other, someone clawing at me in the middle of the night, noises in my ears, could not cry was numb, extreme dizziness, nausea, insomnia. After 4 years, still feeling spacy. Over three years, lying around on the couch, could not think properly, had no incentive, isolation, difficulties in socially, could not relate to people. Yes, doctors, how arrogant, egotistical, incompetent, monstrous of you to ignore your patients who many times just want somconc to talk to, to be validated. Automatically pull out that pen and prescription pad, "yes, we know what will fix you, we will give you a tablet" that will calm your down, make you numb, keep your brain in limbo, masquerade your feelings, keep them hidden out of sight, we are used to giving out pills, that is what we do, medication will help you. And we know about side effects; all medications have side effects; but the good of medication outweighs the bad. "We have given you something, we have done what we do best, and we have fixed your problem." Many say they receive no cutbacks from the pharmaceutical companies, all those free samples, writing pads, calendars, coffee mugs, travel benefits, and what else? So you completely screw up my brain so it was upside down, every day trying to gain some sort of equilibrium. Having no energy, no initiative, disinterested, trying so hard to valiantly stay afloat, being embarrassed because of lack of motivation called laziness, gave up on my poetry writing, artwork, just wanted to sleep, bright lights, loud noises, harsh smells, seems like my mind was all twisted up, like strings of Christmas tree lights all tangled, desperately trying to keep alight, when the electrical impulses were delayed, detoured, weak, fragmented, nothing ran smoothly, nothing lit up all at once in unison, some were lit, others never fired, never gave a glow. I walk around like a zombie, afraid to make any abrupt movements fearing that I might just splinter into pieces and be blown away by the least bit of breeze.

I am only one in thousands of people, and even very young people whose lives have been changed, and, not for the better, some people have even more horrendous effects from being on certain drugs, and end up ending their lives, or ending others. Doctors are inept in treating patients in the adverse side effects of medication especially in withdrawal, have no idea, and then prescribe other drugs to minimize those side effects. It is imperative that doctors need to be further educated in withdrawal/weaning from medication. It is all very complex I know, and prescribing drugs upon drugs without the overall health of the patient long term is not taken into consideration, fixing the problem now, can often lead to more severe problems later on without careful monitoring."

—From Petition Ref S

"In July 2003, at the age of 45, I experienced my first major depression. I started taking 40mg. of the antidepressant Paxil a day. By September, I was feeling mentally healthy again. After forgetting to take Paxil for a few days in February 2004, I weaned myself off the drug. I started to feel depressed again in July. My symptoms included insomnia, increased anxiety, rapid weight loss, low concentration and a lack of energy. I put myself back on 40mg of Paxil a day.

A few days after I started taking Paxil again, I was having suicidal thoughts. I thought I could get rid of the thoughts and recover more quickly if I increased my dosage. On July 17, I started taking 60mg. of Paxil a day. Three days later, I planned my suicide. I went from planning my suicide to planning a murder-suicide to planning a murder. On July 31, 2004, I killed my 11-year-old son Ian. I was charged with first-degree murder. In November 2004, I was diagnosed by one of the leading forensic psychiatrists in the world as being in a "major depression" with "psychotic episodes" when I killed Ian. In May 2005, his assessment was supported by another leading forensic psychiatrist, who was hired by the crown attorney. On September 30, 2005, I was judged to be 'not criminally responsible on account of a mental disorder' for murdering Ian. I received an absolute discharge from the Ontario Review Board on December 4, 2009."

—From Petition Ref QQQQQQQ

"I cannot include most of what happened to me whilst taking and coming off the prescribed antidepressant as it is too traumatic for me to revisit. My life has been destroyed by taking a prescribed antidepressant. Serious side effects and adverse reaction was not picked up by doctors. My mental and physical health deteriorated over the three years I was on it and it all came to a head when I hit tolerance. My body and brain just could not tolerate the drug any longer and hell broke loose and I lost any kind of a normal life altogether. I am a mother to two children and a wife to my wonderful husband who; if it wasn't for them I would not be here. The symptoms and experiences I have had to endure as a result of taking a prescription antidepressant have been inhumane and most of it -I couldn't find words for. My children have lost their mother in so many ways. I can no longer function like I once did -physically and mentally. Most of my days are spent lying down on the sofa or in bed because the pain, exhaustion, fatigue, head pain or depression is too much. I suffer cognitive problems which affect me in so many ways. I lost my emotions altogether—I cannot feel love, happiness or any good emotion. No connection to life. I have become sensitive to chemicals, foods and have been advised to stay away from all prescription drugs as they would have a negative effect on me. I have had to endure psychosis, suicidal depression and suicidal urges. The most horrific mental torture one can imagine. I would never have thought those states were possible. I can no longer exercise which is something I loved to do prior to this ordeal. I have lost friends and any kind of social life. It has been devastating for me and my family. I cannot believe what my life has become. I believe if my doctor had been aware of the dangers, informed of adverse reactions and long term use dangers this would not have happened.

There was no informed consent when he gave me that first prescription. I believe if I had been told, I would never have touched them. I had anxiety induced stress from being in a stressful job, a mother to two young children and having a husband who worked away from home. I was still a happy, healthy young women with a life ahead of me. Now I have no idea what my future holds. I am nearly four years off the antidepressant and still have no signs of recovery. We need to be believed, validated and supported. We didn't ask for this. No one should ever have to go through what I and many others have. Please help this happen. Many other lives could be saved and many helped. Thank you for taking your time to read this."

—From Petition Ref PP

"I had no experience with psychiatry till the birth of my second child. I was admitted to hospital in a state of crisis. My family doctor had not understood the development of my postpartum depression. She prescribed an SSRI which, with any exploration, would have been counter indicated for me. The immediate outcome was a suicide attempt when I jumped at a subway train after ten or twelve days. Twenty three years later I still need a wheelchair, an accessible home, so very many other things as well. I consider myself lucky because I got to be a stay at home mum. I did live. Not everyone survives. I understand from various research resources that suicide is an unsurprising outcome from SSRIs. I believe that SSRIs need to be eliminated. I do not like psychiatric drugs, however I do use them. They slow me down, cloud my brain and interfere with my life. But I am alive."

—From Petition Ref BB

"I have been severely harmed by being prescribed an SSRI at the age of fifteen for situational anxiety. I tried to withdrawal ten years later with severe withdrawal and as most doctors do not recognize withdrawal my dose was increased and I had to continue taking it. Fast forward another ten years and I was co administered another drug for an infection and developed serotonin syndrome and severe side effects. I have been diagnosed with neuroleptic drug induced akathisia and extrapyramidal side effects from Zoloft.

Zoloft has completely destroyed my life. Since this drug interaction two and half years ago and the continued side effects of this drug I have gone from working and studying to being completely incapacitated. The medical profession have absolutely no idea about the severe side effects caused by these drugs or withdrawal. The only solution they seem to have is increasing the dose or prescribing more drugs."

—From Petition Ref FFF

"For those of us who did not suffer from immediate adverse reactions from taking these drugs, many go on to inflict the chemicals into their body and brain while they live 'something of a life.' During this time, they are shielded, tooled up, protected from the stresses and strains of life (although what they are also shielded from is experiencing deep joy and heartfelt passion that can only be felt from the seat of a person's own authentic emotions). They are numb and impervious to making proper connections with people and as such, this can cause great distress in their relationships and personal life.

A parallel to this that is worth pointing out is that if a person walked into a room of 10 people with a knife, and justified it as a protective measure, he would be considered the lowest of the low. He is tooling himself up where he can cause huge harm to people with impunity and the surety that he cannot be harmed in the same way. Mind altering drugs do a similar thing... a family member told me often that when I took these drugs, I had them in tears many times with the things I'd say to them. This next proverb is one that speaks of the importance of acting independently and deciding your own fate emotionally and spiritually. It indicates how it's important to meet life's challenges head on, the ones that are put at our feet, because they are put there for a reason. Probably because these are the lessons that will equip us to learn the lessons we need to and to become the very best version of ourselves.

The Establishment however, cares nothing about your spiritual and emotional growth... what it does care about is your ability to 'get over it', get tooled up and get back to work and contribute to the coffers! Here is the American proverb by Ted Halpern: "Love many... trust few... and always paddle your own canoe!" I'd rather paddle my own canoe (poorly, even!)—going into waters that are less than comfortable, and encountering the people and experiences that will teach me the lessons I have to learn, so I can become the best version of myself—than have a drug pusher strap the chemical equivalent of a jet engine onto my undercarriage, ripping the hull to shreds as I tear through tranquil waters and have them call me a medical success story.

My father died when I was 14. Shortly after this, our 16 year old beloved family dog died in front of me without any chemical euthanasia while I was in the house alone. It took about an hour for him to die. I was transfixed yet traumatized at the same time. A year and a half later, I split with my childhood sweetheart who I'd been with for 2 years; I was a teenager, hormonal, with a sensitive disposition.

There is no record of ANY of this in my medical notes, yet my memories of this time are vivid. The next 30 years were spent numb, insulated but functional, other than when I forgot/stopped/or tapered the drug."

—From Petition Ref GGGGGGGG

"Our daughter Catherine died in November 2010; she was 29. She was given a cocktail of psychiatric drugs over a period of 5 months and sadly took her own life. She experienced adrenal exhaustion after returning from a 6-month world trip in April 2010. She had jet lag and had been only getting 2 hours sleep a night for weeks. Her wedding in Greece was to be the 2nd of July and she had a breakdown 2 weeks before we were due to fly out to Santorini.

There were many stressors also besides the wedding preparations. Catherine was diagnosed with MS in January 2009. She was given Benzodiazepines initially for anxiety and then prescribed Escitalopram for the anxiety and to help her sleep but that's when her nightmare began.

After being on that drug for just over 2.5 months she had bought weed killer with the intention of killing herself. We requested—and Professor Andrew Herxheimer kindly wrote—a report for the coroner. From my understanding of his report, 'escitalopram and its almost identical predecessor citalopram are linked with suicidal ideas and behavior'. And that in his conclusion, 'We cannot ask Catherine what made her kill herself, but it is very possible and even likely that her suicidal thoughts and feelings were induced by aripiprazole and mirtazapine. Their effects would have been additive.'

More and more drugs were added. It wasn't till after she died that we began to find out about the drugs which Catherine was taking. We realized soon after, that it was probably the cocktail of these powerful mind changing drugs that lead to her death. Drugs Catherine was taking prior to her death on 24th November 2010 were: 1) Aripiprazole 20mg mane, 2) Mirtazapine 45mg nocte, 3) Procyclidine 5mg tds, 4) Haloperidol 5mg mane and 10mg nocte, 5) Diazepam 5mg pm to tds, and 6) Zopiclone (as needed).

We undertook research about these drugs. The more we read, the more we were shaken, with ultimate anger building inside us. All she needed was rest and sleep. Professor David Healy has highlighted the adverse reactions to some of the drugs in his open letter to coroners in general. Before the inquest, I received a report prepared by the expert witness from the coroner. The main emphasis seemed to have centered around Catherine's MS. He concluded that MS was the main factor in Catherine's depression and suicide. He claimed that she had an MS relapse. Professor Scolding, who was Catherine's neurologist, confirmed that Catherine never had a relapse. In fact, all the claims made by the expert witness about her MS were totally rejected by Professor Scolding, who is an expert in his field of neurology, and who was also treating our daughter. The expert witness was giving his opinion about Catherine's MS, which is a neurological condition, yet he was contradicting Professor Scolding's opinion, who is an expert in neurology.

The expert witness never saw or met our daughter and I find the claim, that it was the MS that made Catherine depressed and have suicidal ideas, astonishing. However, Professor Scolding did see Catherine, and said in his letter that he was 'always impressed by how well she seemed to adjust to the disorder and by her courage and strength of personality.'

Our daughter was a highly intelligent girl, she was loving, kind and gentle. She always showed much concern for her family and friends. She loved life and was looking forward to her future. Catherine had no history of depression or any mental health problems at any time in her life. She was always upbeat and determined and showed such a lot of courage even after the diagnosis of MS. It was totally alien to her to think or even contemplate suicide. The expert witness in his conclusion cited the key findings from a paragraph from "CSM Expert Working Group on the Safety of SSRIs 2008". It states that: 'There is no clear evidence of an increased risk of self-harm and suicidal thoughts in young adults of 18 years or over.' The report was published in 2004 and not 2008 as he claimed. It is out of date because that finding no longer applies. In 2008, new trials were carried out to show that it now extends to 25 years and not 18. In effect, he reproduced a finding that no longer applies. I personally find this misleading.

At the inquest, I challenged him on this but he insisted it was 2004. He appeared flustered. The expert witness report also stated: 'On 1st November, the dose of aripiprazole was doubled to 20mg when she was last seen by the psychiatrist. It was felt that she was improving.' This was contradictory to our observations of our daughter. Catherine was deteriorating and she was thinking about suicide. The team was contacted on Friday, the 29th of October 2010, and this was pointed out to them. This was after Catherine visited a police station with the delusion that she thought she did something wrong. It is unlikely that the following Monday (1st November 2010) she would have improved. Indeed, my wife was staying with Catherine at the time. There was certainly no such alleged improvement. In fact, quite the opposite: I saw Catherine on 13th November and I was shocked to see how much she had deteriorated. She was agitated, shuffling as she walked. It was evident she had akathisia. Akathisia is the extreme inner restlessness which can be caused by antipsychotics and antidepressant drugs. The affected person feels tortured from within and these drugs can contribute to or directly cause or lead to suicide.

On the morning of the day Catherine died, she had an appointment with the Early Intervention Team. They had knocked on her door, received no reply and left. No precautionary attempt was made to contact someone which would have aroused suspicion that something was wrong. Depending on the time involved, this may even have saved her life. Indeed, Professor Herxheimer informed me that in his opinion, the level of care that Catherine received was INADEQUATE. I pointed this out, together with other detailed responses that I made about the expert witness report. I wrote and sent two lengthy and detailed reports to the coroner.

They both took extensive time and research from various sources, including articles written by experts who are at the fore front of pharmacology research of these psychiatric drugs. Both of my reports were also discarded by the coroner. The coroner continued and made a despicable verdict of suicide. We were hoping for a narrative verdict. After the inquest I wrote to the MHRA, who published 'Report Of The CSM Expert Working Group on the Safety of SSRIs.' Indeed, they confirmed it was 2004, thus showing that the claim made by the expert witness, which he emphatically defended, was wrong.

One drug that Catherine was prescribed was escitalopram, which the expert witness gave his opinion on. At the beginning of the hearing, the coroner's officer, when reading out her report, said that Catherine had a history of depression. I was taken aback but too upset to respond to this. I had lots to think about and I was certainly not accustomed to court hearings. I made it clear that prior to June 2010, when Catherine had a breakdown, she had no history of depression. When someone says this person has a history of depression, one immediately envisages many years. This is totally false. So what was meant by 'she had a history of depression?' I wrote a letter to the coroner pointing out all of the above, together with evidence. She wrote back and said she couldn't comment on the points I raised, and that her decision remained.

In summary Professor Herxheimer and Professor Healy have jointly written a paper titled 'Case Histories as Evidence,' which has been published in 2012 by International Journal of Risk & Safety in Medicine. It explains how it is that many courts have not adequately considered prescribed drugs as a cause of death which I believe to be a very sad state of affairs."

—From Petition Ref AAAAA

"I was prescribed an SSRI antidepressant in 1996, at the age of 41. I went to the doctor complaining of intermittent insomnia when I was away on business, plus PMT. I came away from the consultation with a diagnosis of being on the edge of a 'clinical depression' and clutching a prescription for a drug which I was assured was not addictive. I was absolutely not on the edge of a nervous breakdown (I had to look up the meaning of clinical depression) and Seroxat turned out to be most definitely addictive.

However, when my doctor stated these facts, telling me I had a chemical imbalance in my brain (also untrue), I believed him absolutely. Dr. David Healy, in his book 'Pharmageddon,' describes how in the mid-90s, the drug company marketing teams were telling doctors that, for women, a critical marker for depression was insomnia. Seroxat was the new non-addictive solution, rather than a short course of sleeping tablets, which is how this problem had been handled up to then (and what I was expecting to be given).

Instead, I ended up with a strong neurotoxic drug which has damaged my health—complete overkill for the problems I presented. This has happened to many people, particularly women. What followed was years of trying to stop the drug and failing. At first, I thought I was terribly ill with a major anxiety disorder. Eventually the penny dropped that I was experiencing withdrawal, which each time I stopped the drug would give me symptoms of insomnia, anorexia, indescribable anxiety, phobias, the list goes on. There was never any formal acknowledgement from my doctor that withdrawal existed or agreement that that was what I was experiencing. My only recourse was to take the lowest dose I could to keep the withdrawal at bay. I had to keep taking it in order to function.

In 2008, I was found to have osteoporosis, a side effect of Seroxat as noted in the patient literature. In 2009 I developed a movement disorder. I lose voluntary control of my body and jerk violently as if I am having an epileptic fit, although I am awake. It is deeply unpleasant. This is considered by the neurologists I have seen to be either Medically Unexplained (MUS) or a Functional Neurological Disorder (FND). Most I have seen will not engage with me in the possibility that nearly two decades on an SSRI could be the cause. One neurologist was enlightened enough to consider it as an option and agreed to refer me to Dr. David Healy in North Wales, who is an expert on SSRIs and Adverse Drug Reactions. His diagnosis was clear and immediate on hearing my story—an ADR between Seroxat and Alendronic Acid (for osteoporosis). He has seen the same movement disorder due to the same ADR in other patients before and since.

In 2013, I decided I had to stop the drug, whatever the withdrawal consequences, in the hope that if I did the movement disorder might stop too. I have been through four terrible years of indescribable withdrawal symptoms, and I am coming out the other side. I now have a dysfunctional nervous system, I still have the movement disorder, and I have a dysfunctional digestive system which prevents me from eating a number of foods or taking any supplements or drugs. My nervous system responds to any drug I try to take by making me jerk violently.

Where government funding is going at the moment seems to be purely into drug misuse services. There is no recognition at policy level that patients who have become dependent on drugs which were taken wholly in line with their GPs prescribing guidelines require a different approach in order to withdraw from these dangerous neurotoxins. It is exemplary that society puts so much money and effort into helping people who misuse street drugs.

However, we who did nothing other than believe our doctors and follow their advice deserve better than to be expected to line up at a drug misuse center and be counselled to come off a benzo or SSRI in the same manner as one would a street drug. It can take months or even years, depending on the length of time it has been ingested, to withdraw from a prescribed benzo or SSRI.

It is imperative that appropriate tapering guidelines become available UK wide. My experience is, and my expectation continues to be, that any time I need access to NHS services my issues are distorted by the view that I took an SSRI for 17 years in total and therefore I have a history of 'mental illness' which affects my physical health. What I want is for any nurse, doctor, specialist, or consultant to look at my records and say, as a matter of routine, 'yes, after long term use of an SSRI your physical body has been affected at a number of levels and we need to take that into account when treating you.' Please help us get that level of recognition within the medical profession. Our experience is that they don't want to know, they don't want to believe us and 'it's all in our minds.' Again, I will say—we deserve better."

—From Petition Ref ZZZ

"I have had anxiety from a young age but always tried my best to carry on with things. I completed school and was working. But as I got older my anxiety got worse. My problem, and what caused my anxiety was bowel issues. I was scared of needing the toilet when I went out. This led me to avoiding places and would go out at certain times when traffic wasn't bad so I could get to my destination at a quicker pace. I went to the doctor about it as I was starting to have panic attacks and knew I needed some kind of talk therapy. This was never offered to me and the medication 20mg citalopram was given, I was told to take it every day. No warnings about side effects or withdrawals where given.

After about a year spent on 20mg, my anxiety didn't change, it was still there but I kept taking it in hope that it would work eventually. After a year had passed I went to see my doctor again and was told to increase to 40mg. Over that year on the 40mg my anxiety increased and got worse. I also developed a slight tremor and the panic attacks were more frequent and longer lasting. This then started to interfere with my job. I was a care worker for adults with autism and challenging behavior. I loved my job but part of it was taking them out to do activities. I struggled continuously with panic attacks one after the other. I then could not cope and went on to night shifts so I didn't have to go out anymore. Went back to the doctors and was swapped straight onto sertraline/Zoloft 100mg. Nothing got better it just kept getting worse, I was dizzy all the time my migraines were constant; life was a mess.

I went back to the doctors and was then put on to the highest dose of 200mg. I stuck this out for another year with nothing getting better, just getting worse, but I listened to the doctors that it was just my anxiety. By March 2016 I had had enough; I had to quit the job I had been in for the last 8 years, my life was a mess, my body was a mess. I had constant tremors and migraines and I had now gained another illness on top of it all—agoraphobia. I was petrified of going out of the house because I was so scared of my panic attacks by this point. I went from a girl who would have anxiety when having to go on long journeys to a girl who had panic attacks over and over again in my own home.

March 2016, I spoke to the doctor again and was swapped onto 15mg of mirtazapine. Taper schedule was only a month from 200mg of sertraline. I began to take the mirtazapine and after about two days I started to feel very restless in my body but I kept taking them as I knew it takes a while to get into my system. After nine days my eyesight went and my whole left side of my body went numb like I had been given anesthetic. I thought I was having a stroke or a heart attack. After half an hour it got no better so I rang the paramedics. They came out and did an ECG and told me everything was ok but they would like me to go into hospital. I couldn't as my agoraphobia was that bad; I could not leave.

After a while my eyesight came back but I was still completely numb down my left side. The following morning, my face was still numb but I continued to take the mirtazapine for 5 more days. As the days continued I became more restless internally and felt very dizzy and numb. I phoned the doctor again and they told me to stop them and go on to 20mg of fluoxetine. After the very first dose I could not keep still I was pacing the house day and night in a constant panic attack, what felt like adrenaline coursing through my whole body. As the days went on it got worse and worse I was convulsing and twitching I didn't sleep for two weeks straight as every time I tried to go to sleep I would be jolted awake and would have this compulsion to pace. Fourteen days I lasted on the fluoxetine, and I was petrified to put anymore in my body. I stopped and did not take anything after that. It has now been 10 months since this point and it has been absolute hell; my body is a complete mess. I have had these symptoms constant for the whole 10 months and it doesn't seem to be getting any better:

- Constant tingling all over my body, especially worst when I first wake up and when I'm trying to sleep. Feels like I'm plugged into the electric.
- Akathisia, cannot sit still, an electrical current running through my body 24 hours a day every day. I pace back and forth around the house as I cannot keep still.
- Burning skin, like somebody is holding a match under my skin at all times, yet my hands and feet are numb and cold.
- Bloated beyond belief.
- Dizziness; I don't know what it feels like to not feel like I'm on a rocking boat in the middle of the ocean.
- Itching, like there are millions of bugs on my body. Sometimes it feels like they are trying to get in, sometimes it feels like they are trying to get out.
- Body jolts, most annoyingly at night when I'm trying to sleep. It's like some annoying farmer is prodding me with a cattle prod.
- As soon as I eat, it feels like my body goes into more dark places; anxiety levels increase
- Small amounts of food send my blood sugars up from 5.5 to anywhere between 8 and 10.
- Absolutely petrified to eat anything too sugary.
- Urination approximately 4 times in an hour every hour. Bladder always feels full and heavy.
- Body temperature always low (34.9°C) even though I don't feel cold.
- Clenched jaw all the time that then gives me headache. Acid/ firework feeling in my head with heavy pain.
- Stabbing pains all over me.
- Anxiety is on another level that I never had before.
- Crying about 20 times a day.
- Heart palpitations.

- Pressure in my head like my nerves are rubbing together.
- Blood pooling in my legs and feet, when I stand up my heart rate goes to 150bpm.
- Jump out of my skin by the slightest noise.
- Ear pain, heavy buzzing, feeling constantly.
- Akathisia, pacing, shaking, twitching, cramping just pure hell and torture.

I have had no support from the medical community and just told over and over again that it is anxiety and I need medication. The medication never helped me and just made my life a complete mess. I am very ill and I'm 29 years of age. I should be out there enjoying life but I'm stuck bed ridden in pain."

—From Petition Ref NNNNNN

"I would like to submit my account of attempting to withdraw from the SNRI antidepressant drug venlafaxine (Effexor). I am a 42 year old woman. I have taken the medication exactly as prescribed and have never abused it. I was prescribed the drug by a psychiatrist to treat depression and anxiety after other medications had been ineffective. He explained I would need a high dose as one of the active ingredients was only effective then. I eventually ended up taking 375mg a day of the drug. I took it for several years.

In 2016, it was decided I needed to come off the drug because of side effects developing. The plan had been for me to withdraw over a period of a few weeks. The first few reductions in dose were difficult with brain zaps (a feeling of electric shocks in the brain) and zaps throughout my whole body when I walked. I would also experience bizarre and vivid dreams, nausea and night sweats. I needed to leave a lot longer than the psychiatrist recommended between drops as those symptoms lasted for around a month. I was told I could reduce in dose every 2 weeks. When I got to later doses, the withdrawal symptoms become intolerable, with my mental health deteriorating as well as the physical symptoms.

After reducing from 37.5mg to half a 37.5mg tablet my depression got out of control. I experienced uncontrollable rage which is completely out of character for me and included me screaming and shouting at people. The worst rage ended up with me kicking and throwing things around and then stormed out of the house in a deeply suicidal frame of mind. I drove past some woods and then had the idea of hanging myself and drove to the 24-hour supermarket to buy rope. Instead I sat in the car park thinking of ramming my car into things before phoning someone.

It was after this meltdown that I saw my GP. Her response was to increase the venlafaxine again, which would have just made withdrawing harder in the long term. I ended up needing to take a second antidepressant drug to help with the symptoms of withdrawal. I feel like I am stuck on this medication now. Whenever I am late with a single dose I experience extreme brain zaps and more worryingly twitchy eyes which makes me worried I am going to have a seizure. Doctors do not recognize how bad antidepressant withdrawal can be for some people and instead dismiss their symptoms or attribute them to a return of depression. They tell patients to withdraw too quickly when the brain and body needs time to adjust to changes in medication after long term use. I have had to turn to the internet to find out more about how to safely withdraw from venlafaxine and my psychiatrist has now prescribed liquid venlafaxine and is allowing me to taper very slowly after me showing him information I found online. It should not be up to the patient to research their own symptoms and find their own cure. What happens to the patients who do not have that information to hand?"

—From Petition Ref VV

"At the age of 35, I became pregnant with my third child and to the outside world (and to me) my life appeared straightforward. But I had a secret: a secret that I had managed to hide since childhood, and a secret that I shared with only one other person—it was a secret of abuse, and the consequences of sharing this secret with anyone else would be devastating (or so I was led to believe) and whenever I contemplated it, sheer terror would engulf me and I would feel overwhelmed. So much so, that I remained silent—or rather, I was silenced, and so I buried that secret deep within me, in the hope that it would over time disappear. But it was not to be, and I wonder sometimes, how I ever thought it would disappear.

The birth of my son in December 1996, proved to be the moment when this secret reared its ugly head and shortly after his birth, I found myself in need of support to manage my distress. Believing that I could trust in the expertise of professionals, I turned to statutory mental health services for help. I was immediately prescribed an antidepressant for my symptoms and so began a journey that was to last 17 long and at times desperate years. By November 2013 I was sicker than when I first encountered mental health services. I had become one of those infamous revolving door patients, been given five different psychiatric diagnoses and had lost all sense of personal responsibility for my own well-being. I was dependent on doctors, nurses, locked wards, cocktails of medication (anti-depressants, anti-psychotics and mood stabilizers) and ECT. I began to self-harm by cutting and burning myself, I abused alcohol and smoked cannabis. I attempted to take my own life on more than one occasion, and I'm sad and ashamed to say that at one point I wanted to take my own children's lives as well as my own.

Unfortunately, throughout all those years, I never felt safe enough nor was I able to find someone who I trusted enough within statutory services to disclose the horrifying nature and cause of my distress. I had lost not only those 17 years of my life, but much more; those first precious years of my children's lives and the final years of my parent's lives had passed me by without my noticing and to this day, I have scant if any memories of my children as they grew up and of my parents as they grew old, became ill and sadly passed away. By this time, my spirit felt completely broken and I had simply become a label—a set of numbers from the Diagnostic & Statistical Manual of Mental Disorders. I hated myself and the life I was living.

I felt disempowered, dehumanized, re-traumatized, hopeless, isolated, afraid, ashamed, guilty and angry but most of all, desperate. I believed the time had come for me to leave the world for good and I put together a plan—I chose the method I would use and the place where I would spend my final moments. I did my best to write a meaningful letter to each of my children in an effort to explain my actions. I organized my finances so that my family would not have to worry about the cost of funeral expenses and I wrote a will dividing up my estate.

But the warrior within me wouldn't allow me to carry out my plan. On the 6th November 2013, it was decided that I should come off, overnight, the cocktail of psychiatric medications I had been taking for 17 years, and my world was turned upside down. Whilst this rather brutal decision was made for me and I had no choice in the matter, it proved to be a momentous turning point in my life. I was totally unprepared for what was to follow, as were my family and friends and the following weeks, months and years proved to be incredibly challenging and at times agonizing. I experienced unimaginable emotional upheaval, anxiety and insomnia so debilitating I was at times unable to function, I cried when I didn't want to cry, I laughed when I didn't want to laugh and I felt intensely angry when I didn't want to feel angry. I experienced moments of utter despair, moments of sheer elation and moments of paranoia. It felt like my brain was constantly working on overdrive and I found it incredibly hard to sit still, I felt compelled to be doing 'something' all the time.

Whilst some of these experiences have improved, I am still experiencing difficulties with sleep, agitation and anxiety. I cannot compare the experience to anything else I have ever lived through. However, challenging the process has been and still is, I don't regret being taken off all medication—to remain medication free has been one of the best decisions I have ever made in my life, because now, despite all these withdrawal symptoms, I am "living" and not just "existing". Now when I walk down the street, I look up at the sky and I notice the world around me. My curiosity, passion and zest for life are evolving day by day and I can sometimes look in the mirror and smile back at my reflection. Now I am emerging as a person capable of feeling, facing and coping with every human emotion it is possible to experience, and that feels so good. I now have hope instead of utter hopelessness. Now I feel empowered and have choice and control back in my life. Now I am finally beginning to find a true sense of self and purpose. And four years later, I continue to remain drug free. I haven't seen a psychiatrist or been in contact with statutory mental health services for over 2 and a half years. I am living independently in the community surrounded by my family and friends and coping with everyday life."

—From Petition Ref GGG

"My citalopram nightmare: At the age of 28, one month after my birthday, my life would change as I knew it. I went to my GP after my honeymoon in 2014 and decided to come off citalopram. I was no longer experiencing anxiety and was desperate to lose weight and eventually start a family. My GP's advice was to come off the drug over two weeks. I did as my GP instructed, reducing the dose in half and alternating daily. I experienced some mild head zaps and some morning anxiety I was unfamiliar with; however, this soon disappeared.

Fast forward 18 months off citalopram, I experienced some anxiety and stress having moved home, town and needed to find a job. The stress of applying for jobs, attending several job interviews, and financial worries bothered me, so I went back to my GP. Within a few minutes I walked out with a prescription for citalopram in my hand, the standard 20mg therapeutic dose, believing this would help the stress I was experiencing. What happened next is unimaginable to most people, and for my family and me, truly heart breaking. After a couple of days back on citalopram I was delusional and psychotic. I thought I had murdered my husband and dog with a kitchen knife. I believed I was a danger to everyone, and had nonstop intrusive harming thoughts, no sleep, no appetite, pains, severe agitation, and an episode of hypomania (elated, thinking I had cured anxiety). This went on for about eight weeks. During those weeks I was informed by GPs and staff at the local hospital to stay on citalopram and would soon find myself on a cocktail of citalopram, lorazepam, diazepam and quetiapine.

I was deteriorating, losing my mind as my brain was being chemically tortured by these drugs, my poor body unable to metabolize them. I knew these drugs would kill me if I didn't get off. Symptoms of drug toxicity had already began when my GP performed blood tests whilst on citalopram. Blood and urine tests revealed I had very low potassium levels in my kidneys (requiring 2 ECG's), raised blood counts, and protein and ketones in my urine.

I came off all drugs on 1st August 2016. I desperately hoped I would be back to my old self and the six-week hell of an ordeal would be over. Only that didn't happen. It's January 2018 as I write this email to you. I haven't felt a positive emotion since the reaction. I battle suicidal thoughts daily, purely because I can no longer identify with who I used to be. I am a shell of who I was. I suffer with chronic fatigue, severe apathy, serious episodes of depression, depersonalization/derealization, unable to sense time or atmosphere, racing thoughts, poor memory loss, unable to form new memories, confusion, vivid dreams and nightmares, blurred vision, visual snow, and tinnitus. There isn't a moment when I am symptom-free. My life is now in ruins. I want to assure you I never experienced any of these symptoms prior to this citalopram and would never have considered myself mentally unwell. I had never seen a psychiatrist. I had a normal life as a wife, worked full time in financial services, enjoyed hobbies such as swimming and cooking, could drive and enjoyed holidays. I now have to live off disability benefits and live in council housing because I am unable to work, and my marriage fell apart last year.

What I would like most from this is for the medical community to stop informing patients these pills are safe and effective. Inform patient's why suicide is a side effect and what can happen if you are unable to metabolize these drugs. Health care professionals to be more aware of the symptoms of serotonin syndrome, withdrawal and neuroleptic malignant syndrome. Monitor patients closely beginning antidepressants. Work together in the medical community to produce safe tapering plans for patients wishing to discontinue antidepressants. Please take our accounts seriously. I assure you if this happened to you or someone you know you would do everything in your power to see these drugs only prescribed in desperate measures and would want to prevent this happening to anyone else. How many more lives are going to be taken and damaged needlessly?"

—From Petition Ref QQQQ

"I was physically injured from Lexapro (escitalopram) and Xanax (alprazolam). I am disabled in ways that are still hard for me to even grasp. These medications destroy much -needed receptors in our brain. Without them we are unable to function on a human level. The things I have experienced are pure torture and there is no help. People are committing suicide just to make the pure terror and pain stop. It's inhumane what happens to us. And the doctors do not even recognize that this can and does happen. We are left alone to try to survive this. It has been described as human torture chamber.

I am 10 months out from taking these medications (poisons). I was a happy and very productive women. It was given to me for a thyroid condition. And has destroyed my life and my brain. I have central nervous system damage. Pain like no one should have to live with and akathisia, cortisol rushes, agoraphobia (never was afraid of anything!). I have not been able to leave my home since. I have lost everything!!! I even lost my ability to speak or walk when this first hit. It's a horrific injury caused by these dangerous drugs. I never abused anything. Took as prescribed!!!! There are people taking their lives because of this. Not because they are crazy. But because the torture is unbearable. I don't know if I am going to survive. Please help us."

—*From Petition Ref FFFFFFFF*

"'What symptoms did you experience?' I am on day seven of my second attempt at a reduction and missed the deadline again, because of the wall climbing feeling of wanting to get out of my body. I can't sleep as every time I close my eyes the spinning vertigo feeling exacerbates my nausea... then every inch of my body feeling weighed down by something makes my breathing labored, a lack of oxygen making me feel panicky and shortens my breathing to the point I feel anxious and hyperventilate... this is not fun. To have all of this on top of my issues?

'Were you warned about the withdrawal symptoms?' No one told me it would be like this. I was told I would be weaned off. No one told me that a doctor's advice (reducing my venlafaxine from 300mg to 225mg) would find me laying in the street (2016 my first attempt at coming off venlafaxine). I had strangers call a paramedic who then threatened to slap me as she stated I was not having a panic attack, but I was having a tantrum!

'Were you believed by doctors when you told them about the side effects?' No, no, and definitely NO. Only one doctor took on board what I said, unfortunately I have since moved and no longer have her support. A paramedic empathized completely as she herself went through the experience!

'How has your life changed since taking psychiatric medication?' Downhill, don't work, bored, and unable to do anything productive. I'm very debilitated by this antidepressant. This is such a good opportunity to share with people: professional people, the government, about the horrors of taking psychiatric medication. So we don't want to miss this opportunity to share as many horror stories about psychiatric drugs as possible, as so many doctors don't believe us!"

—From Petition Ref DDDD

"In 2016, after 15 years of having medically undiagnosed symptoms which left me chronically fatigued, often dizzy and just generally feeling ill often, I was finally diagnosed with a disorder of the nervous system called Postural Tachycardia Syndrome (PoTS). For 7 years, the only treatment I was given was an antidepressant to up my energy levels and probably to treat what doctors thought was actually anxiety because of my dizzy spells. Although I was never diagnosed with depression, my GP at the time told me antidepressants often help with energy levels and dizzy spells and weakness.

Whilst being referred to a cardiologist to rule out POTS, my GP told me 'that dose of antidepressants is so low you may as well not take it or up it' so when I got my POTs diagnosis, I tapered my dose for a week or so and then stopped taking it. Although I have always been highly sensitive, the only thing which had made me feel genuinely low for long periods was dealing with my hellish fatigue and symptoms and being told I was 'FINE'.

I don't berate that GP as she was the only one who sent me for any further testing in 15 years, but I believe she was just following the current guidelines for withdrawal which are not helpful for most people. After around a month off the meds although I was on a high from my wedding, I soon started to feel a little odd. I was having strange dreams and crying in restaurants over small things, I also was seeing very odd scary images in my head.

And then I lost a beloved member of my family, and was crying daily, feeling like a dark cloud was following me. I just did NOT feel OK and I did NOT feel like myself anymore. My GP said it was nothing to do with withdrawal; that it was just grief. Yet I could see images of the holocaust in my head and just felt like I was in a constant state of fear. I had NEVER experienced anything similar in my life.

I still to this day do not know 100% if I was having a withdrawal or grieving badly, but from talking to other people, I believe a lot of what I experienced were withdrawal symptoms. It was VERY hard not to go back on the tablets and I am deeply sorry that I had to feel like that during the first 6 months of my marriage. I only wish my GP had told me to slowly wean off my medication so as not to suffer as I did. As a trainee psychotherapist who has had 4 years of long term therapy with two different therapists, I am sure this was out of character for me and that a lot of my symptoms were due to withdrawing from citalopram."

—From Petition Ref VVVVVV

"Eighteen years ago, my 12 year old son was prescribed Prozac (fluoxetine) for depression. Not long afterwards, he was found dead in the orchard next to our home. His death was initially determined to be a suicide, but later when an attorney examined his autopsy report, he called for the investigation to be re-opened as a possible homicide. My son had been with a friend on the day of his death, and his friend had also been prescribed an antidepressant. Three experts provided statements indicating that homicide should not have been ruled out, and that the initial investigation had been poorly done.

I am convinced that my son's death was the result of dangerous drugs prescribed to two adolescent boys whose parents were never provided with enough information to make a truly informed decision about whether the drugs were safe or not. I testified before the FDA in Feb 2004, demanding that SSRIs be removed from the market, or at the very least have the strongest of warnings be placed on all SSRI drugs. The warnings finally came through later that year, but they came too late for my son.

These SSRI drugs are not safe for everyone. There is ample research that indicates a small percentage of people cannot properly metabolize some of these drugs, but when you consider that millions of people are taking these drugs, that 'small percentage' translates into tens of thousands of people who are likely to experience adverse effects that far outweigh any benefit they might receive. It's time to stop supporting drug companies who lie and hide crucial evidence and to protect the citizens of your nation against harmful drugs!"

—From Petition Ref NNNNNNNN

"I suffered a very bad reaction to antidepressants that made me so ill that I lost 15 months from work. I took an SSRI antidepressant for the first time in my life aged 40 after I was experiencing some mild anxiety for a few weeks. I went to see my GP who gave me sertraline. I took it that morning and by 5PM I had started to vomit and had the first panic attack that I had ever experienced in my life. By evening I had started to feel not only depressed but started to have strange thoughts about committing suicide by hanging myself. I did not realize that these medications could cause all this and thought I had suddenly gone mentally ill in a few hours.

I went back and saw another GP, crying, very distressed as the sertraline had given me insomnia, too. The GP gave me a new antidepressant to try (fluoxetine) and diazepam to help me sleep. Within a few days I had become much worse. I could not sit still, sleep, vomiting constantly. I began to hear voices and asked my husband to take me to hospital as I felt extremely suicidal. I went to hospital, where I was told it was lack of sleep causing my symptoms and was to continue with the fluoxetine and diazepam and was given some zopiclone sleeping pills and the crisis team began making home visits.

After another week, I continued to get worse and the crisis team doctor agreed with me that I was having a rare reaction to SSRI antidepressants after I refused to take it anymore. I was put on a new sleeping pill called trazodone to help me sleep. I did not realize that this was also an antidepressant. This was in March 2016. My GP increased the dosage without asking me. I could not tolerate the higher dosage so tried to come off the antidepressant and ended up in A&E again with electric sensations. Crisis teams were called again and the doctor thought the dosage changes had increased my anxiety, so he lowered the dosage and added another pill (pregabalin) for my anxiety on top of the trazodone and diazepam.

I became so ill my GP sent me to a mental health center (secondary mental health services). They added another antidepressant (duloxetine) to all the medications that I was taking. By this time, the crisis team had a CPN nurse visiting me also. A few days into taking these medications I was seen by the crisis team who wanted me to go into hospital as they thought I had the strangest case of post-natal psychosis they had ever seen as it does not usually come and go.

I now know that I am sensitive to not only taking these medications but also to starting and stopping them and dosage changes. I was in hospital for six weeks. I felt even worse when I got out but had got used to feeling suicidal. My doctor kept me on the trazodone after I refused to carry on with the other medications apart from diazepam. He added another pill called buspar. I began to get problems with my neck and face muscles and in February 2017 was pulled off the medication cold turkey. Ten months later, I'm able to work again but still have a problem with my neck muscles and electric sensations. These medications caused me to lose two years of my life but am hoping to fully recover. I have now been signed off from mental health services."

—From Petition Ref RR

"I believe I have been damaged by psychiatric drugs. All told, I spent over 30 years on a variety of different antidepressants such as Anafranil, Seroxat and Effexor. In 1979, my marriage was failing and I was seven months pregnant. During this distressing period in my life, I was referred to psychiatry.

It was at the suggestion of my psychiatrist that I started on Anafranil, one of the older tricyclic antidepressants, after assurances it was safe in the last trimester of pregnancy. As it turned out this was not the case as my baby had convulsions at 8 hours after birth, directly attributed to withdrawal from maternal Anafranil. My psychiatrist was unaware this could be a problem. Many studies now seem to suggest that there is an increased risk of autism spectrum disorders in taking antidepressants in pregnancy.

In hindsight, I wish I had never taken an antidepressant. It should have occurred to me to come off them but I had been diagnosed as having a depressive illness and I thought I needed drug treatment. This, I feel disempowers the patient from seeking non-medicated routes to solving their problems. Paradoxically as the years progressed antidepressants did not appear to improve my health. Most days it was a struggle to get out of bed. It was becoming clear to me that antidepressants were causing me considerable problems. Any time I failed to get my prescription I felt panicked and jittery. The side effects were debilitating and wide ranging. I was plagued by blurred vision, heavy sweating, fatigue, irregular heartbeats, weight gain, photosensitivity, hives, gastrointestinal problems, deficiencies in memory and concentration and a general feeling of apathy. I had no motivation beyond taking my pills and dragging myself through the day. There were times when I ended up in hospital after failed attempts to come off antidepressants without appreciating I was actually in withdrawal—something none of my doctors ever picked up on.

I would have liked the help of my GP to taper off my antidepressant but I knew he preferred I take them indefinitely. I hadn't anticipated having any problems coming off Effexor if I kept to a reasonable taper plan, though in retrospect I wish I had prolonged the taper for far longer. I thought I might have some difficulties for a few weeks, perhaps a couple of months at most, as I'd once been told, but the idea that withdrawal might last years seemed inconceivable. Initiating a taper in 2010 was my chance to regain my health after many years of feeling chronically unwell, but had I been aware that I risked suicide and years of protracted withdrawal symptoms I might have thought twice. Nothing in the medical literature ever prepares you for the brutal experience many of us face coming off psychiatric drugs, antidepressants included.

Within a week of being off Effexor, I had terrible panic and inner turmoil on a scale I had never encountered before. I was crippled by this constant torture that I rarely left my sofa beyond going to the bathroom. I lived minute to minute. I barely slept or ate. This was a nightmare that had no end. I tried desperately to reinstate antidepressants but with no success as they made me feel much worse. During this time, I had a psychiatrist tell me I needed antidepressants like a diabetic needs insulin. In the summer of 2012 I attempted suicide.

Without the help of my family I would not be here today. After a short spell in a psychiatric hospital, I was discharged with a prescription for yet another antidepressant alongside Valium and a sleeping tablet. I had failed to convince my doctors that I was suffering from protracted withdrawal; instead my symptoms were seen as evidence of relapse. Life was unbearable and I was prepared to try all sorts of treatments that in other circumstances I would never have considered like Seroquel (an antipsychotic), Pregabalin (a mood stabilizer) and benzodiazepines. Thankfully, I had the resolve to say no to lithium and ECT.

Because doctors/psychiatrists are largely uneducated about antidepressant and benzodiazepine withdrawal, patients run the risk of further unnecessary and damaging psychiatric drug treatments. Polypharmacy increases the likelihood that patients remain stuck on these medications for life with implications for their health."

—*From Petition Ref C*

"I am writing in support of this petition as this is the supposedly civilized thing to do in a civilized, democratic, accountable society. But let me tell you there is no civility or accountability in the gross harms many have suffered because of psychiatric drugs. Also, what good are elected representatives if the issue is never addressed but is repeatedly brushed under the carpet?

These drugs have wrecked my life, both on them and after withdrawal. What is worse I should never have been on them in the first place as my problems could and would have been resolved eventually. What sort of treatment thinks that prescribing dangerous drugs hardly tested and with unknown effects is going to help anyone? Without wishing to sound like a conspiracy theorist sometimes it seems that mass drugging of the populace is a desired outcome as the same thing happens again and again. Antidepressants, benzodiazepines, amphetamines, barbiturates, opiates, cocaine the list goes on. For over ten years now I have suffered from the most horrendous symptoms every second of every day with no relief at all. I have been left unemployable, I had to give up studying as a part time mature student, lost relationships and have had any semblance of normality obliterated.

I am lucky in that I have a good GP who is prepared to listen and who has been receptive to literature on this subject, but it still is no real help as nothing has helped at all with these symptoms. I still suffer from screaming tinnitus, insomnia, pins and needles all over, burning down my spine, pelvis and down my legs into feet, akathisia, intense anxiety, panic, drug sensitivity, chemical sensitivity i.e. paint fumes, gastrointestinal issues, bladder issues, apathy, weakness, jelly legs, faintness, tingling, suicidal thoughts alien to myself and more. This is torture and every day is a struggle to survive.

Prior to these drugs I was a healthy 28 year old man but now, twenty years later, I have been robbed of everything. And for what? Certainly not any supposed benefit. Whilst taking them I was a different person, irritable, angry, aggressive, paranoid, violent, uncaring, insensitive and I nearly lost my family, friends and my life. Now people can see the real me again and they are in agreement that those drugs were the cause of my personality change. I began drinking and smoking heavily and taking drugs although I never touched street opiates as I had still some sense to know the outcome of that addiction, but ironically opiate withdrawal is over in a matter of weeks whereas psychiatric drug withdrawal has lasted over ten years.

Due to my behavior, I was arrested four times and spent time in prison and I have this stain on my character for life. Much more happened whilst under the influence, yes I use that term the same way as alcohol as that is what these drugs are, not medicines but mind altering drugs. I am so angry about what has happened to me and countless others and any right and just person should be equally outraged. This is a scandal on a grand scale and one that needs to be brought into the cold light of day. How much is it costing the public purse, my estimation countless millions as I have estimated just myself running into hundreds of thousands of pounds when you add everything up. Drug costs, doctor visits, specialists, hospitals, prison, probation and social security benefits as an example. How is this allowed to happen? It needs to addressed and addressed now."

—From Petition Ref XXXXX

"There are far more problems with these prescribed psychotropic medications, such as antidepressants and benzodiazepines, than without them. There is nothing really wrong with the human condition, being sad, angry, traumatized by life events. It's our body's natural response to life's difficulties. But our bodies are equipped to recover, given time, patience, understanding, acceptance, practical help, as well as nudges from non-pharmaceutical interventions such as exercise, relaxation techniques, acupuncture, meditation, mindfulness, talking therapies, being in nature, etc. There's an endless list of non-pharmaceutical possibilities. My life was deformed by prolonged use of antidepressants and benzodiazepines. Not once did any medic suggest I might be better off without them. I was convinced by this 'therapy' I was an inherently bad person, and I would always need their poison to 'cure' me. The longer I stayed on them, even though it was a 'low dose', the more paradoxical the effects of them became.

Well, I'm not inherently bad, I'm just a normal human being, so please don't anyone at all rewrite my reality. I'm left with a very poor memory and cognitive impairment, balance issues, musculoskeletal problems, muscle wastage, and many other withdrawal symptoms.

When I reflect on how much I suffered through out my life from both side effects of taking the poison, and now with protracted withdrawal symptoms, I can only grieve for future generations who will likewise suffer if this pharmaceutical propaganda is allowed to continue."

—From Petition Ref FFFFFFF

"I am submitting an anonymous submission for the purposes of bringing to light serious emotional/psychiatric harm sustained by taking antidepressants, and the side effects that remained even after discontinuation. I'm a 30 year old female and I've had PSSD (Post-SSRI Sexual Dysfunction) since 2009. I have a history of severe OCD and began taking brand Zoloft when I was 16 to treat my symptoms. I had no sexual side effects at all but ended up tapering off the medicine when I was 20 because I could no longer afford to pay for the medication. After I discontinued, the OCD thoughts came back, and three months later I was on meds again—only now I was taking the generic sertraline, at the same dose, because that was all I could afford without insurance.

I became asexual literally overnight. I lost all genital function, had no ability to reach orgasm, no sexual attraction or fantasies whatsoever—it was like a switch had been turned off. The prescribing psychiatrist told me this was normal, though, and to stick with the drugs, which I did for a few more months, until finally I got fed up and 'cold turkeyed' off the medication. Even though there were no longer any drugs in my system, every single side effect remained. For the last nine years, I have tried almost everything I can think of to get my sex drive back. With a few, temporary exceptions, nothing has succeeded in giving it back to me. I have taken all kinds of herbs/pills and done all kinds of exercises. I even took Bupropion XL, which delivered very inconsistent results and unfortunately gave me a seizure. Nothing has truly helped.

Right now I am involved with a community of similar PSSD sufferers called the PSSD Forum trying to find answers and hope. 'Did your doctor warn you about the withdrawal effects?' My psychiatrist did not warn me about any side effects. After starting the medication, when I brought up the fact that I did experience side effects, he said that it was "normal" and to continue the medication. When I abruptly discontinued the medicine, the side effects remained. No one was concerned about it except for me. Subsequent doctors and psychiatrists I visited—including a gynecologist—told me that it was normal for a woman to have a low sex drive, and that I shouldn't worry about it.

'Have pharmaceutical drugs harmed you?' The loss of sex drive has been devastating to me. I no longer feel desire, arousal, experience lubrication, or have orgasms. My genitals feel 'dead.' I still have OCD, but without taking the medication that harmed me, I have no way of treating it. 'Have you had to give up work?' I have not given up work. However, the self-loathing and lack of confidence I felt after my fallout with the medication was life-altering. I no longer felt like a woman or someone that anyone could love. As a result, I 'aimed low' in life, turning down opportunities to better myself and be happy. I avoided social situations out of shame. I also allowed friends and family to treat me badly, telling myself I deserved no better because I wasn't really human anymore.

My doctors told me that it was depression and OCD that made me feel this way, not loss of sex drive. I was frequently told 'there's more to life than sex' and to not worry about it, even though I was in a loving relationship with someone else, someone with a disparate (healthy) sex drive to mine, and we used to have fulfilling, uncomplicated sex on a regular basis. Nine years of PSSD have done much to tear my life and mental health apart. Thank you for allowing me to tell my story. I hope it helps others."

—From Petition Ref HHHHH

"In March 2015 I went to my company doctor with work stress. I did not meet the ICD-10 criteria for depression at all. I had no problems getting out of bed, was not suicidal had no increase or decrease in appetite. I was just stressed and not sleeping enough due to long hours at full time work and in my part time studies. My doctor, in a 5-minute consultation and without explaining anything, handed me a prescription for venlafaxine. Venlafaxine is a third choice antidepressant that is normally prescribed for treatment resistant depression. It was the first antidepressant I ever took. The pharmacy filled the prescription of 10 pills without explanation and without handing out the patient information leaflet.

I took this medication for five days and got several dangerous side effects, one of them severe bleeding; aside from that agitation, insomnia, paranoia and more. After five days of horrendous side effects, I stopped the medication according to the doctor's instructions. Aside from feeling hungover, I was completely fine for a day. Until after about 36 hours the withdrawal symptoms set in. I suffered convulsions, myoclonus, urges to commit suicide, rapid mood swings, aggression, crying, sweating so much that we had to change the bedsheets 5 times per night, involuntary movements, tremors, passing out, vertigo, dizziness, arrhythmia, chest pain, vomiting, severe suicidal depression, paranoia, anxiety, electric shocks in the brain, disorientation, cognitive problems, memory loss, concentration problems. The list goes on and on. I had over 70 different, disabling symptoms.

I got no help from my doctors. Due to the extreme involuntary movements, my neurologists diagnosed me with a 'functional movement disorder,' migraines, and chronic fatigue syndrome. I had none of these issues before taking and stopping the venlafaxine. I was off work for 2.5 years due to these symptoms.

To this day, I still suffer severe symptoms. I had to return to work because I cannot afford to have no income. Disability payments were denied because a 'Functional Movement Disorder' is, in the views of the neurologists, not enough grounds to be off work. They ignored the other symptoms I have and generally disbelieved me. I am at work now, trying to survive every day without getting fired. I have to leave meetings often because I get seizure-like episodes. I forget simple instructions and have to sleep often during the workday. The drugs have completely eradicated the ability to feel any positive emotion. They have practically made me inhuman, only able to feel negative emotions or numbness. I feel disconnected from the few friends I have left after being 'mysteriously' sick for years. Before, I was always an overperformer at work. I had many friends. I was a person other people enjoyed to be around. Now I'm a shell of my former self, constantly in agony, electric shocks shaking my brain every couple of minutes, feeling numb and disconnected. I feel let down by the medical profession who poisoned me, denied the harm they caused and refused to give me any help or support."

—From Petition Ref GG

"At 41 years old, I entered perimenopause with a resounding thud. The cluster of symptoms I presented with to numerous medical professionals, all pointed perfectly to menopause.

Despite a family history of early menopause, and all the symptoms that suggested menopause, I was refused hormone treatment due to being too young to be going through menopause. And so my journey to beyond the depths of hell commenced. I do feel it necessary to point out that prior to the drugging that would ensue, I was an extremely highly functioning member of society.

I never suffered from anxiety or depression, I had a near perfect life and I woke up every day reminding myself how lucky I was to be blessed with such a wonderful life. But that was suddenly about to change when benzodiazepines were introduced to combat menopausal insomnia. From the very first benzodiazepine pill 3.5 years ago, I have lived in a tortured and altered state of reality. I took benzos for approximately four months during which time I was in and out of the doctor's office, pathology, emergency department and specialist offices. My mental and physical health declined rapidly. I could not function and was bedridden, my family holding a bedside vigil as I prepared to say goodbye to my family. My family and I had no conclusion to reach other than an obscure undiagnosable disease that would ultimately led to my death. Having no answers and deteriorating rapidly, I was then cold turkeyed off the equivalent of 20mg of Valium and put on the antidepressant Effexor. I took this drug for two weeks, during which time I openly started talking about suicide to the husband whom I loved and adored, the father to my young children whom I loved and adored.

Shortly after my introduction to Effexor I hospitalized myself and was diagnosed with major depression. Never at any point did any medical professional suggest it could have been the drugs despite there being mounting undeniable evidence that should point in that direction. The horrific symptoms that I encountered during this time (some still to this day even at 16 months off the drugs) are too numerous to list, but here I provide a small sample for your reference: suicidal depression, akathisia, extreme anxiety, brain zaps, amnesia, lack of any human emotion aside from extreme fear, intrusive thoughts a human brain would not normally produce, inability to differentiate hot from cold on my skin, visual disturbances, paranoia, hallucinations, olfactory hallucinations, hearing loss, nausea, optical migraines, severe vertigo, tinnitus, myoclonic jerks, extreme nerve pain, inability to cry, feeling detached from reality.

These symptoms are unforgiving and beyond cruel. What is even more distressing than these symptoms is the fact that every second person I speak to is on these drugs, or has been at some point. Often they have been put on them for depression when all they wanted was counselling. They did not believe they even had depression. They continue to take them not because they are ill but because the withdrawal symptoms are life threatening both physically and mentally. None of these people have been warned of the addictive nature of these drugs and thc horrific withdrawal symptoms which can last years, and nor was I. How can the medical establishment and governments continue to ignore the damage these drugs are causing? Suicide rates are increasing, depression is increasing and so is the prescribing of these drugs. If the drugs worked rates would be decreasing. How can this simple fact be ignored? Prescribing of these drugs must stop.

Withdrawal centers for psychotropic drugs must be established along with support services. Please take notice of these submissions, and act accordingly. This is an epidemic which is responsible for the deaths of a number of innocent victims. The family members of people who have committed suicide on these drugs, and due to horrific withdrawal they cause, need to know the truth about why their family member died. The world needs to know the truth."

—From Petition Ref MMMMMM

"I am a mother of three. As of today, I am seven months and eight days clean off my antidepressant venlafaxine (Effexor), which is in the SNRI group. I am still very much suffering from after effects and in recovery after long-term use. Which means today I am not able to tell my story to the best of my ability so I will give you the bones as best I can. The main reason I want my story heard is that after I was manipulated and coerced into taking this drug, I was told it was not addictive. I was essentially just left on the medication for years; this stretched eight and a half years. They did not make me better.

The beginning is probably a common story. I had a difficult time at home and at the age of 18. I was diagnosed with clinical depression. After I left home I was signed off work and given various medication. But there seemed to be a lack of education around it; I was not offered any counselling or even any information regarding the medication itself. I was left with a packet of drugs with no warnings or support. I will admit to not taking to them properly; I took one or two and they made me sick so I went back and said they didn't work so was sent away with different ones. But in my mind, I thought they worked like a painkiller; that they should work instantly, and they didn't.

When I was 20, I had my first daughter and things changed. I thought I'd turned a corner and I look back at that young woman and feel utter sadness and regret and dearly wished there was proper support and understanding for young people dealing with issues. Like most young woman with troubled backgrounds, I suffered with post-natal depression. By the time my daughter was 10 months old I had lost too much weight. The doctors told me I had to stop breastfeeding and if lost any more weight I was going to be sectioned.

This is where the story gets difficult. I had a very clear ultimatum. I had no family around me and a partner who had no clue how to do anything let alone look after a child. I was seen by the mental health team who were urging me to put things in place so if I was sectioned, I would need to have someone to legally care for my daughter. The pressure was on me to put on weight and one of the nurses persuaded me to try the venlafaxine the doctors were trying to prescribe. I felt manipulated as I wanted to find and alternative but with no other option I took them. There I believe my fate was sealed.

The following year I fell pregnant again, this time with my partner ending the relationship if I went ahead with the pregnancy. I couldn't not have the baby so then not only did my relationship breakdown, the doctor told me I had to discontinue the medication. Of course I knew this but I was extremely vulnerable! The doctor told me he would give me a week half a dose and that was it. I said to him, 'Could we please not do it too quickly?' He looked at me unsympathetically and sniggered, 'You aren't on crack.' Of course, I won't be the only person that says that this drug is addictive.

I went through hell, but I did have a baby and a baby on the way to suffer through. I was suicidal and agitated which I was never before. I was repeatedly told it was not the medication. My home life did improve after this; I settled down with another partner and although still vulnerable to past issues I was able to function, get a job and my weight was stable. I then had my youngest daughter who was born just as my middle daughter turned two. I breastfed her for over a year and was quite happy. However when I stopped breastfeeding, the cracks began to show: I felt low, tired and tearful. I went to the doctor, a different doctor but another one who looked at just one solution. I was put back on the medication.

What follows is a train crash and the end of life as I knew it. The medication made me detached and unable to focus on normal day to day activities. Four months later, we moved home and my daughter was admitted to hospital with meningitis, and although I was able to focus on getting through the initial crisis. I had a complete breakdown. I became increasingly suicidal, anxious and agitated. My dosage on my antidepressant was doubled and I was given valium and sleeping tablets. This concoction of drugs given to me seems baffling to me now as I was openly saying I was suicidal but it was followed was a cycle of uppers, downers, increased agitation and psychosis. I became manic and reckless; I felt more and more detached from reality. The medication was open to abuse and I started to abuse alcohol to calm down or quiet my mind.

For nearly three years I had a range of professionals walking in and out telling me I was ill and I was not doing enough to put it right, I needed to work with everyone. Great things to say to someone who is agitated and suicidal. I was however repeatedly asking for help. At one point I was at the doctors at the very least once a fortnight but sometimes on a weekly basis asking for help. At no point did anyone address the issue of medication or even query it. After a particular bad episode I tried to come off the tablets. I was put on a lower dose. I stopped any other medication.

Things within my home life began to settle so I started to stabilize around it. I don't believe I mended; I just started to function better around it. I became less agitated and reckless but I became more detached. In this sense, professionals slowly stopped having concerns, I stopped asking for help, things seemed to get better on the surface. But the issues didn't go away; the tablets still affected my thought process. My memory is patchy and they made me aggressive and volatile. I became a machine and worked nonstop. I feel like years have just fallen out of my head. For the last seven years I've had no break, no way of listening to the needs of my body or life. I stopped feeling anything; I didn't know when I was too tired or too hungry.

After a particular stressful end to 2015, I felt I had to address my life and most aspects. When I was able to reduce my workload, I weaned off the venlafaxine, still believing that they wouldn't be addictive. The withdrawals were utter hell but the shock was genuinely believing that physical effects were all I needed to worry about. No—the utter horror is now months later I am suffering with days of severe agitation sleepless night and debilitating headaches amongst other things. I believe that we all have the right to find out why we were persuaded to take these drugs and why we were left on them for so long. I feel I was manipulated into taking them and then told they weren't addictive and then repeatedly criticized for my thoughts and feelings on the medication. I feel I was let down and could very easily been a suicide statistic and forgotten about. I am not and I will be vocal. But I feel my children were let down repeatedly and were robbed of their mother. I trusted a system that clearly didn't know what it was doing and I deserve to find our whether I have been left with permanent damage."

—*From Petition Ref Y*

"I was prescribed citalopram (an SSRI) for 'mild depression' in 2013, after I messed up my first year in university. Who wouldn't be in a bit of a downer after that? Regardless of context, I was labelled with 'depression' when I was compared against a questionnaire conducted by the GP. I often question after this assessment and the label attached to me of 'mental illness'; at what point is it not normal or not simply being human to express emotion at negative life experiences? Is happiness the only acceptable emotion we should hold in ourselves, regardless of circumstances? If I had arrived there and told them my close family relative had died and I was feeling down about it for quite some time, I can guarantee I'd be told I had a mental illness.

This prescription given to me, it was the first port of call, and no counselling was offered. I had several minor reactions to starting the drug—most prominent of those was being unable to get to sleep for two weeks. I used to walk the streets of my town in the middle of the night just so I had something to do and to reduce my frustration. Other side effects included a stiff neck, stiff jaw, teeth chattering and inner shaking. I was reassured by my GP that these side effects would take six weeks to settle and it wouldn't be until then that I would see the full benefits of the drug.

I remained on citalopram for two years. Within a month of being initially prescribed the drug, a doubling of the dose was made by the GP and I remained on that dose, until one day I questioned, "Why the hell am I taking this?" It served no purpose. I had no follow up or monitoring from my GP who prescribed it. It was as if they prescribed it to me indefinitely. I merely felt a former shell of myself; emotionally numb for 2 years, with no highs and no lows. What sort of life is that? Unable to feel human emotion—a chemical lobotomy."

——*From Petition Ref DDDDD*

"In 2009, my son, who had never been depressed in his life, went to see a doctor over insomnia caused by temporary work-related stress. He was prescribed the SSRI citalopram, and within days he had taken his life. At my son's inquest, the coroner rejected a suicide verdict, but delivered a narrative verdict, citing citalopram by name as the 'possible cause.'

After the inquest, I noticed that what happened to my son was far from unique. Eventually, in 2013, I began the 'AntiDepAware' website. This includes links to reports of inquests held in England and Wales since 2003, most of which have been discovered in the online archives of local and national newspapers. It must be noted that this list is far from exhaustive, but even so, contains over 5,500 reports on self-inflicted deaths, all of which are related to use of antidepressants. As my research continued, certain trends became more noticeable, so that I was able to conclude that the link between antidepressants and suicide is heightened: 1) In the early weeks of uptake or if the dosage is increased, decreased, withdrawn, or changed for another brand (This is highlighted in the British National Formulary) 2) When SSRI antidepressants have been prescribed alongside other psychiatric medication, such as anti-psychotics or benzodiazepines 3) When the deceased has been prescribed antidepressants not for clinical depression, but for what NICE terms "sub-threshold" conditions such as anxiety, PTSD, work-based stress or grief.

Much of my research has been directed towards children who have taken their lives after being prescribed antidepressants. Because of the acknowledged risk of suicidal ideation, NICE Clinical Guideline 28 lays out three criteria, all of which must be met if antidepressants are to be prescribed to children under 18. These can be summarized as: 1) Only if the antidepressant prescribed is fluoxetine; 2) Only if the child has been diagnosed with moderate to severe clinical depression; 3) Only if it can be shown that the prescription has been preceded by at least 3 months of "specific interpersonal therapy" which has proved ineffective. In other words, NICE regards the prescription of antidepressants to children as an absolute "last resort" option. Nevertheless, antidepressants continue to be prescribed to children in ever-increasing quantities, in total contravention of NICE Guidelines.

I have also researched the over-prescription of medication for ADHD. This has been shown to lead to conditions like bipolar disorder in teens, which in turn has been mis-medicated with SSRIs. In 2015, I was contacted by a Human Rights organization, asking permission to use my articles The Lost Children and The ADHD Epidemic as part of a submission to the United Nations Committee on the Rights of the Child in Geneva. In June 2016, the UNCRC published their investigation into children's rights in the UK. Sections 59-62 of the report dealt with mental health. Here, the committee voiced their concerns over the over-medication of children. They reported that 'The actual number of children that are given methylphenidate or other psychotropic drugs is not available,' and that: 'There is reportedly a significant increase in the prescription of psycho-stimulants and psychotropic drugs to children with behavioral problems, including for children under 6 years of age, despite growing evidence of the harmful effects of these drugs.' One of their recommendations was to: 'Ensure that prescription of drugs is used as a measure of last resort and only after an individualized assessment of the best interests of that child, and that children and their parents are properly informed about the possible side effects of this medical treatment and about non-medical alternatives.' Earlier in 2016, the World Health Organization had raised concerns about the rising level of antidepressants prescribed to children in the UK and other countries. I don't believe that the government has made public its response to either the UNCRC or WHO. If prescribers in both the public and private sectors continue to ignore the guidelines published by NICE and the BNF, the numbers of adults and children who take their lives will continue to rise. These deaths are preventable."

—*From Petition Ref MM*

"I was on Prozac 20 mgs for a little over 20 years. I was told by a psychiatrist I would need to take Prozac for life due to a chemical imbalance. When my mother's health declined rapidly, I was switched to venlafaxine (Effexor) being told that Prozac was no longer working. I had MANY debilitating side effects that my psychiatrist said had nothing to do with venlafaxine. I didn't find this out until I missed taking one venlafaxine 150 mg capsule and couldn't walk without hanging on to furniture and walls.

That's when I looked up venlafaxine side effects and was shocked to see all my side effects for a solid year, which I was seeing specialists for, were related to venlafaxine. I was LIVID! Last week of March 2013, I told my psychiatrist to put me back on Prozac. She bridged me, reducing venlafaxine by 50% for 2 weeks and adding Prozac 20–40 mgs for 2 weeks. The first day of reducing my venlafaxine from 150-75 mgs were PURE HELL! I was naive and didn't know anything about withdrawals; no one told me anything. My psychiatrist just told me to go to the ER, where they told me I was going through withdrawals from venlafaxine and sent me home like it was nothing. The ER doctor told me to stay hydrated and crawl in bed. I was shocked that they let me get behind the wheel of a vehicle! I found myself driving on the wrong side of the road driving home, only realizing it when I saw cars driving towards me. Yet when I told my psych doctor I couldn't drive, she told me if I didn't go to the ER she wouldn't write me a note for work.

I came home and crawled in bed still reducing my venlafaxine as told by my psych doctor. I wouldn't wish this on any living being. I had uncontrollable and severe shivering, jerking, sweating, hallucinations and blurred vision, vomiting, diarrhea, dizziness, brain zaps, heart palpitations and racing heart, body wreaked with burning pain, felt like bugs crawling underneath my skin, vivid nightmares, my brain wouldn't work to even form a thought (COMPLETELY disconnected with body and earth). The only thing I could do was endure this hell staring at the wall in front of me. If I closed my eyes I had white dots coming at me. I had a vision, so clear it was like I was there: I was in a crowd of people right after Jesus had been hung on the cross. It felt like my brain and body was shutting down. If I was able to think (form a thought) I would have ended my life and suffering in an INSTANT without a second thought.

This has been the most cruel, mental and physical torture anyone can endure. I went through this alone, bedridden, rarely ate because I couldn't get out of bed, when I did it was SO HARD to nibble on crackers, fix a piece of toast, cereal or microwave soup to eat and everything I ate I either vomited or it went right through me. After going through a hell of withdrawals I knew nothing about, I had a long list of symptoms and was suicidal. Psych doctors kept trying me on multiple drugs (1–4 at a time) only to make me worse for the next 6 months. I finally told my psych doctor that I would only take Paxil 20 mgs (I just picked one) and see what happens, since NOTHING was working. Paxil didn't work either, but I was desperate and felt like I needed something but didn't know how to fix myself and doctors didn't either. I lost my job, family, friends and would've been homeless if it wasn't for my savings over the years.

Out of desperation I made a Facebook group called "EFFEXOR (venlafaxine) Side Effects, Withdrawal and Discontinuation Syndrome" not expecting anyone to join and now have over 3K members. It took me almost a year to figure out what I was experiencing was Post-Acute Withdrawal Syndrome (PAWS), also known as Protracted Withdrawals and the reason I couldn't get any medical help, attention or support is because it's not listed in the DSM-5 manual. My life as I knew it came to a screeching halt in pure torture overnight due to our failed so-called healthcare system and medical professionals. It's been 4 years and 8 months of hell (with numerous debilitating symptoms). Currently, I can barely take care of myself; showering approximately every 3–4 weeks, sometimes longer; can't fix food to eat, pay bills, rarely brush my teeth, etc. I have an in-home counselor that comes once a week for 1½ hours to check on me and help me with things like getting my mail, getting me groceries, etc. My house hasn't been cleaned since all this happened to me. On top of my numerous symptoms, I still deal with my withdrawals which have stolen all my desires, goals, you name it. I feel completely blank inside. If you want a list of current symptoms I can put a list together for you.

All of this could've been avoided if our healthcare system and so-called professionals informed patients; about withdrawals, acknowledged that antidepressants can cause withdrawals and protracted withdrawals, knew how to taper patients slowly and safely off antidepressants (10% or less every 3–4 weeks that I've read about), and STOP prescribing drugs to try and cover up withdrawal symptoms just to name a few."

—*From Petition Ref JJ*

"As a result of taking antidepressants, I now have multiple severe disabilities that include 13 different areas of visual distortion, balance issues, visual processing issues, co-ordination, sleep issues, digestion issues, joint issues, memory issues, a mast cell problem, neuro degeneration/dysautonomia that was diagnosed by a private clinic in London (letters can be produced if necessary), and multiple chemical sensitivity among many other symptoms. The informal dialogue that comes about when a patient is in a doctor's surgery is hugely telling of the lengths that doctors will go to ensure that the patient is guilted into taking responsibility for the situation in which they find themselves.

When I visited my doctor for the umpteenth time only to be told that my symptoms were very complex and a solution was not something he could give me, he said to me: 'I see a great many people living miserable lives, but THEY just get on with it!' I asked to speak to a psychiatrist and said to him (quite angrily which I think is wholly understandable) that they have no right to hijack and dismantle peoples' lives, he responded 'I think you'll find that we already have!' When I asked an earlier doctor what the outcome would be if I were continually prescribed stronger and stronger medication (as was happening), he leaned back in his seat and told me the name of the mental health ward at the local hospital. When my brother-in-law voiced his concerns to my GP that he didn't know best how to help me, as I was tapering Effexor, and that I was hysterical and paralyzed with fear when he (my brother-in-law) spoke at length with me during the night on the phone, the GP responded, 'She has transferred her dependence of the drug onto you! If I were you, I'd put a block on your phone line so she can't call!' The psychologist who saw me for 2 years and stated firmly to my GP in a letter that he believed my difficulties were of a physical origin and not psychological. When he retired from his position, he shook my hand and said to me, 'You do realize, don't you, that your life has changed forever?'

Perhaps the most stunning words or gesture I've seen is when I went to the Scottish Parliament and spoke with Scotland's Minister for Health and Wellbeing along with one of the principal medical advisers to the Scottish Government. I recounted a horrifying account that spanned 10 years of symptoms that were unimaginable to most people. It was obvious that at a humanitarian level, they were moved and empathized deeply with the challenges that I have been given. At the end of my dialogue, expecting everyone to get up and leave, the adviser leaned across to me, brought their head down to my level, reached for my hand, shook it, while they looked into my eyes and said, 'I'm so very sorry!' This is where I struggle: clearly this was a personal apology and not a professional apology.

People need to understand how this can be the case that harms can be done, apologies can be given, yet for them... this is an end to the matter? Why is this? Because their lives haven't come to an end! Well it doesn't come close! It doesn't even begin to cut it... not for me, and not for the many thousands of people who are and have been harmed week in, week out, year in, year out!"

—*From Petition Ref RRR*

"I want to speak firstly about how when I first realized there was a huge problem that the apparent 'neglect' would show itself and the good doctors would have all hands on deck saying stuff like: 'There's a really big problem here... somethings very wrong... one of our patients has become disabled in many areas of her functioning... and all that's happened is that she took a drug under our care, under our instruction and with trust in our word that it is safe! We need to look into this because clearly something's gone wrong!'

Fast forward 10 years, and I'm still waiting, locked in a reality that I don't want to be in! The whole idea that doctors have been simply neglectful is long since gone from my vocabulary! How stupid was I for thinking that my doctor would be saying to themselves that it is morally, ethically and medically wrong to turn a functional person into a disabled person even if they experience sadness and from time to time anxiety. It's worth mentioning here that any sadness or anxiousness I experienced was as a result of external stimulus! Which is wholly human and completely understandable.

Now, however, there is no chemical stability inside my body! Whereas before chemical stability was something that I took for granted! What staggers me beyond words is this: All these mind altering drugs are just what it says on the tin! Mind… Altering… Drugs!!! So why then, when a patient has taken these drugs and they are in a state of suffering clearly tortured by the legacy, do doctors think it's okay to raise their eyebrows and imply to the patient that this suffering is the patients fault? Geez!!! The drugs are targeted DIRECTLY at the brain and the workings therein!

As doctors keep schtum throwing in a few medical terms for good measure, friends and family look on in astonishment not knowing what to make of behaviors that sit totally at odds with the person they have known! It's been said that the lie is never in what you ARE told by your doctor—it is in what you are NOT told! This would ring true, because it appears to me that doctors smugly assure patients that the drugs are safe to take and what I believe they fail to tell patients is that the drugs are not safe to stop! That little nugget doesn't become apparent to the patient until they try to come off the drug. By which time, the resultant behaviors/symptoms/legacy is medicalized as a separate condition requiring? You've guessed it! More drugs!!!

I remember the words of someone who worked at the Council for Information on Tranquilizers Antidepressants and Painkillers (CITAP) who said 'Imagine you have seen a color that is a totally new color that has never been seen by anyone before only you can see it! How would you go about ensuring your description ensured your friends, family or colleagues could also see it?' The problem with this is that no matter how hard you would try, it would be pretty much impossible for them to 'get it!' Why? Because, they have no point of reference for it; they've never seen it before, so any known descriptors are of no use to them!

Equate this to a person's neurochemistry being messed up with the drugs! The carnage left behind has affected all of their bodily systems. Psychologically they feel distanced, weird, messed up, disturbed… all of the above, and their actions and behaviors reflect what they are experiencing internally! Again, I come back to the previous example. Unless you have experienced this, how can friends, family and colleagues possibly relate?

This inability of family, etc., to relate to these challenges suits the state to no end! All they have to do is shrug their shoulders, throw around a few random labels that they made up (honestly, it's true!) and do nothing and allow the patient to demonstrate the system's 'original findings' which are that the person has a mental illness.

The evidence against psychiatric claptrap is mounting and will only continue to mount up so that the filth that is known as psychiatry will float to the top where everyone can see it! As for myself, I want to speak about my doctor/patient relationship and how it has manifested over time. My doctor's practice has asked me to leave the practice and go register with another doctor. They have suggested that I register at a practice near a caravan that I spend time in! It's quite an unusual thing to happen given that my home is 250 yards from the practice. The lengths that the establishment will go to remove discomfort from their line of sight is astonishing.

I want to finish up with a quick summary. Nearly a decade off these drugs, still severely disabled, I have major visual disturbance in 13 different areas of my vision. Burning/stinging/crushing pains in my skull 24/7, ice packs needing changed every 20 minutes for the last 10 years, balance issues, memory issues, digestive issues, cognitive issues, sleep issues. I'm still waiting for my two week withdrawal to come to an end and wandering in the long grass looking for a doctor, having been told to go elsewhere."

—*From Petition Ref YYYYYYYY*

"In 2000, I experienced pains in my wrist and arm from keyboard overuse in my job at work. I presented to my doctor for a prognosis. I want to make it clear that at this point in time I had never experienced any kind of psychological distress neither was I emotional. The doctor told me that I had a pain in my arm because I had a chemical imbalance and that I needed to take a series of medicines until I found the right one for me. Having never smoked, drunk or taken any kind of drug, legal or illegal, I asked if these were addictive. I was told no, they weren't. I asked if they had any side effects. I was simply told maybe you might experience a dry mouth. I did not know that these drugs were used for psychiatric purposes.

I was given a sequence of drugs to take to heal my repetitive strain injury in my hand, amitriptyline, nortriptyline, venlafaxine, and clonazepam. I worked my way through these medicines over several months finding they were no use and then quit them. Several months later, I start to experience uncharacteristic emotional manifestations. I started to experience unusual crying spells and had what I would describe as my first ever kind of panic attack. I didn't even know what a panic attack was. I presented back to my doctor and said that there was something wrong with me but I don't know what it is. I was immediately given a prescription for paroxetine assured it was not addictive and no side effects, there was no clinical assessment done of any kind. I cannot for the life of me understand how it came about but I stayed on this drug with several failed attempts to quit it until January 2010. The doctor just simply kept renewing scripts all of this time. No discussion was ever had on getting off this drug.

In January 2010 I told him I wanted off and was told, 'Okay, just take as much paroxetine as you like.' In other words, just cold turkey it. I knew this was not correct and left frustrated yet determined to break free of this so-called medicine. After a nine month self-calculated taper, I was in a very dark place and presented reluctantly back to the doctor to get answers for what I now know was horrific withdrawal symptoms. The doctor seemed unaware of withdrawal symptoms (or didn't want to know) with coming off paroxetine. On trying to describe these symptoms, I was told I had an underlying depression. I had never used that word before and replied, "That is not correct." I was referred to a psychiatrist. The first thing I said to the psychiatrist was, 'Are you aware of any issues with people coming off paroxetine.' This was his reply: 'If there were issues with people coming off paroxetine, people would be suing the drug companies.' I interpreted this as no there were no issues with people coming off paroxetine so the problem must be myself. My inner conviction told me this was not correct, either. I left determined right then and there not to engage with the medical profession again. I was on my own.

The next few years were the most difficult of my life. The mornings were pure hell. Forget trying to hold down a job each day was a struggle just to survive. Uncontrollable restlessness uncontrollable psychological and emotional distress, sobbing and suicidal ideations were the norm daily for the next few years. I would be the last person in the world to commit suicide yet I consider it a miracle that I'm still alive. It wasn't until in my seventh year of being drug-free that I was able to return to work on a part-time basis. I was unable to pursue my sports passions during this time also. I used to be a top level amateur badminton player. I'm now in my eighth year of being drug-free and trying to pick up the pieces and get on with my life.

I'm unable to sleep with any regularity am seriously sexually damaged and my beautifully trained tenor opera voice has been taken from me. I now find it very difficult to sing and extremely tiring when I try. So much so that I have completely given up this prior passion. It has been stolen from me. I have a very deep sense of being hoodwinked and betrayed by the medical profession. I'm also outraged and heartbroken that I can now see in hindsight that I was made a drug addict by stealth trapped in a mind numbing anosognosia Kafkaesque world for almost a decade!! It is totally unacceptable to me that SSRI drugs are being prescribed, they should be banned. It is totally unacceptable to me that doctors do not acknowledge withdrawal symptoms of these drugs which for some people like myself can last for years.

Any attempt to get answers for the withdrawal trauma results in intelligence insulting labels and comments from doctors. Doctors should be deeply ashamed at their stupidity. And of the life altering harm they are doing to innocent, trusting people."

—*From Petition Ref FFFF*

"I apologize that this may be upsetting to read but I am in such a bad condition three years after an adverse reaction to Prozac. To recap, the adverse reaction felt like something had fried in my brain, taking with it connections to life past, family, interests, personality. It feels like my whole sense of self is gone, and in its place there is this black hell in my head. There are so many mental and physical symptoms that are beyond human endurance. I endure every minute something even worse than the worst suicidal depression I ever had (with hindsight, always in antidepressant withdrawal) and what a struggle that was. I have already spent 16 years battling antidepressant side effects and withdrawal (misdiagnosed as relapse) and doing what I could to try and manage the condition that the NHS had caused but which very kindly then gave me no coping strategies.

This condition from SSRI adverse reaction is way beyond what I experienced as depression or anxiety in SSRI withdrawal. I am only 35 and I'm hysterical often because I feel pushed to end the only life I was given. People that are ending their lives from SSRI withdrawal or reactions are being pushed to literally jump to escape unimaginable agony. Make no mistake about it, this brain torture could not exist naturally. I would like to say more about how doctors and other health care professionals have responded to my assurance that the drugs caused this. A GP got really angry with me and she thinks it is all psychosomatic. It feels like a chemical has burnt and is continuing to burn my brain. This acid burning brain is common in SSRI reactions. An occupational therapist said, 'Even if it is a brain injury, there is research that people who can maintain a positive mental attitude do better.' How can I be positive if I have something that is even more intolerable than suicidal depression? So, the focus goes back to the patient who is like this because they are not doing enough to 'help themselves.'

I went to my most recent GP appointment to ask specifically about the protocol on prescribing antidepressants. I asked the doctor if by prescribing an antidepressant, they think they are correcting an abnormality in the brain. She did not answer me directly, just that these drugs are complicated and that is why patients need to be monitored. And that the risks and benefits would be explained. But it is clear from our petition that even if patients are monitored the adverse effects side/effects are not being recognized. And I was never told that the condition I am in now could happen. When I asked if patients were given other options before antidepressants, the GP said that talking therapies would always be offered alongside antidepressants. My question is, 'Why are talking therapies not tried first?' Her exact words were, 'If a patient wants an antidepressant, then we will give one.' Where else in medicine would someone be prescribed a drug because they 'want one?' And all the while she was interrupting me to ask, 'What about psychotherapy?'

There is a letter on my file from a psychotherapist saying they did not feel they could help. The doctor also said, 'Even if it is a brain injury, people can still live a life.' And what about volunteering, keeping busy? I was busy when I was first prescribed an antidepressant. I struggled and struggled for 16 years keeping busy but with the adverse reaction to the second drug there is no way I can do this. I have had to give up the few things I had left in life. I struggle to see family with the severe distress I'm in and out in public even more so. I don't think there are any more adequate words in the English language to describe what I have. All I can say is it is torture. The NHS definition of depression is 'unbearable sadness.'

Screaming because it feels like something is being drained from the brain causing something so low no human should have to experience, I don't think fits the NHS description. It is very strange that when I tell doctors something has happened in my brain that I absolutely cannot live with, the response is, 'There are things you can do to help yourself.' They know that I'm on the edge of suicide every second of every day and if they could feel it they would absolutely know the drug caused this.

I am absolutely certain no anxiety or depression could ever feel like this, so this leads me to wonder on what basis are these drugs ever prescribed? If someone is suicidal? I'm severely suicidal from the drug; now I'm being told that I can 'help myself.' If someone as bad as me could deal with their condition naturally, then surely these drugs shouldn't have a place at all. Of all the years I have spent in and out of crisis centers for withdrawal induced depression and anxiety, one nurse said to me, 'You just have to keep trying things and hope someday you will find the answer.' What is so shocking and astounding is that all these years I felt so uncomfortable on the drugs and every time I tried to come off them, neither I nor my doctors knew I was suffering from withdrawal effects and so clearly the answer was not going to be found in anything other than the drugs themselves.

Thank you for reading and I hope this drug induced prescribing hell stops soon before many, many lives are taken."

—From Petition Ref DDDDDDDDD

"I was prescribed venlafaxine by the doctor I was assigned at the Mother and Baby unit for perinatal mental health. I was diagnosed with Post Natal Depression,(PND) and anxiety at three months postpartum. I was referred by my GP to the specialist unit.

I was prescribed venlafaxine because the citalopram I was originally put on didn't seem to be working. I don't remember the doctors telling me anything significant about coming off venlafaxine. They may have mentioned that I would need to taper off it gradually but nothing more. I was not really in a fit state to question the medication I was being given. I trusted the doctors knew what I needed at that point and I do believe it helped me out of a very bad place.

I decided to start reducing my medication after 18 months. I was taking 37.5mg twice a day (the smallest dose tablet available). On three separate occasions over almost a year I experienced what would be described as a relapse but was in fact my reducing too quickly and it too large amounts, cutting up the tablets. This was my only option as far as I was aware and with no guidelines to follow. On these occasions I experienced: insomnia, extreme anxiety, depressive thoughts, suicidal thoughts, uncontrollable crying, complete exhaustion, lack of energy and motivation, anger, headaches, and stomach problems. All things I had NEVER experienced before taking this medication.

After this, I was lucky to have a very understanding GP who prescribed me the liquid version. I then began a very slow 10% reduction, holding for 4–6 weeks each time. But the symptoms were still intense and often debilitating, happening every time I reduced the dose, a wave of withdrawals lasting days, sometimes weeks. Once I began to feel more human again I would prepare myself then do it all over again, I counted 50 times! All done whilst looking after a small child.

In desperation to get off the medication, on a couple of occasions I tried to speed up the tapering by reducing a larger amount or shortening the time spent at each dose. Every time it backfired on me, leaving me with unbearable symptoms unable to function. I honestly feel the process of withdrawing has been much worse than the original PND. Through the process I was 100% sure I no longer needed the drug for my mental health, but I could not stop taking it. I feel the tapering process has robbed me of the past four years as a mother, wife and friend. I hope this helps to getting something done about the problem of over prescribing this drug and the support given to those wanting to be rid of it.

I am thankfully, finally, off this poison. I took my final dose of around 0.25mg in the summer. In total it took me 3.5 years to taper off venlafaxine. For me, I feel let down by the care I have received once I started to taper off the medication. If I'd known how long and difficult it would be I would have started the taper a lot sooner. I would have appreciated more support and understanding from the doctors that originally prescribed it. I understand I am definitely one of the luckier ones, as my GP has been sympathetic and prescribed me the venlafaxine liquid in order to taper very slowly after I had two failed attempts at cutting down the tablets.

I think there must be better support and ways to help patients that want to get off this medication. Instead of just being told that their original health problems must be returning and therefore increasing the dosage, which I have personal experience of. I'm certainly not completely against the use of antidepressants. I desperately needed help, BUT I don't agree how they are sold to vulnerable people, as a quick fix, with no warning of how addictive they are.

You can't expect being on antidepressants to necessarily be a short-term thing, you may be lucky, or like me you may be trapped in a nightmare for years. Do your research; don't take the decision to start antidepressants lightly. There needs to be support for those who want to reduce or stop their medication, at the moment there is zero support in place. The guidelines are incorrect, resulting in people finding it too difficult & staying on them because there is no alternative. I've experienced firsthand professionals telling me that I must be relapsing.

Of course, not everyone finds tapering as difficult as I have. It depends on the drug, the dose, and of course the person. We are all different."

—From direct submission

"I had experienced anxiety, panic attacks and low moods throughout my adolescence, after having been bereaved in my childhood. I was first prescribed antidepressants at age 19. Sertraline certainly boosted me: I felt alive and confident, and able to throw myself into university life, socializing and making friends. There was a kind of hysterical energy about me. I was young, and a student, and I was certainly not taking the drugs consistently at exactly the same time each day, and sometimes missing days altogether. On days and weeks when I felt low, I would double my dosage to give me a 'boost'.

I vividly remember a time I ran out and missed a day or two and was so debilitated by the nausea and dizziness I felt unsteady, had blurred vision when I moved my head from side to side, and walking up the stairs caused motion sickness. This terrified me, but I still didn't appreciate the significance of this as dependence and withdrawal.

At age 21, I stopped taking the sertraline. I quickly started suffering panic attacks and had a constant feeling of doom. I moved out of my shared flat and back home to my mum's, just before my 22nd birthday. At the time, I wasn't aware of withdrawal, but was quite aware I was having a break down. I experienced sleep paralysis, night sweats, panic attacks and a lot of suicidal ideation. In retrospect, now that I know withdrawal, I can see I was experiencing sertraline withdrawal from stopping 'cold turkey' and my doctor should have reinstated the drug and tapered me off it slowly. Instead, I got a new prescription for citalopram and a referral to a psychiatrist. The psychiatrist concluded I had 'treatment resistant depression' (because I had tried two SSRIs) and prescribed venlafaxine, an SNRI which was more sparingly prescribed. I didn't receive any warning, I wasn't spoken to about risks or side effects at all, and I wasn't asked whether I had any plans to have children.

At the time, of course, I didn't have any clue that these drugs were not entirely benign, my experiences had been solely attributed to me and my mental health. Venlafaxine worked miracles. Within two months of this psychiatric assessment, I was at a festival for a whole month working and having fun with friends I'd not seen for the duration of my six month breakdown. Time passed, and these were happy years. I was so scared of what I'd experienced I was cautious of ditching the drugs. I was busy and young, and worked abroad for a year, too cautious to change my medication whilst abroad, I planned to stop taking it once I moved back home. I never intended to take it long-term, but I took it successfully for three years with no idea as to the dependency I had acquired.

Upon moving back at age 25, I moved to a new area and had a new doctor. My prescription was changed; I was put on a cheaper, generic form of venlafaxine, which was quick release. I wasn't instructed to take it any differently and I was only prescribed enough for one daily dose every 24 hours. However, the half-life of quick release venlafaxine is only 8–12 hours so I was unknowingly going into withdrawal every evening. I took it like this for nine months, completely unaware that my new nervous breakdown was caused by my drugs. This was nine months of insomnia, night sweats that soaked me through, rage and violent impulses, suicidal ideation, obsessive and paranoid thoughts. I had moved in with my boyfriend for the first time, and I was horrible to live with; I spent most nights awake and in turmoil, or finally asleep on the concrete floor of the kitchen because I was so hot and sweaty.

Amazingly, my boyfriend started keeping a diary of my moods, and told me he found a pattern. I was okay most of the day, and took a steep decline into mayhem in the early evening. He said he saw in my eyes when I had descended into upset or anger and was unreachable. This is when we looked at my drugs, and understood the meaning of 'quick release.' I feel so stupid now, but both a doctor and a pharmacist wrongly prescribed the medication and how to take it. I consider this gross negligence on their part. This experience not only traumatized me and eroded my confidence in my own capacity to cope, but I now believe that it messed with my nervous system so much by going in and out of withdrawal, that it hyper-sensitized me to the drug and future withdrawal. I've also discovered, through trial and error and GPs having persistently pressured me off of the brand Effexor and onto generic versions of venlafaxine at different times, that I am affected by the change in brand. I've been made aware through my research of the difficulties and differences in the use of generics, which have a negative effect on many patients.

Age 26, I was now back on the original 75mg Effexor brand extended release. I was too terrified of what had happened to me to want to stop taking antidepressants, I was convinced what I experienced was my own madness and I couldn't cope without medication. The rhetoric around antidepressants, and what I was being told by GPs, was certainly that I may need the drugs for life. But I found it hard to stomach that I may be so unwell I would need to be medicated for life, and yet still received no specialist care from mental health professionals, how can a GP decide I need to be medicated for life with no further investigation? A couple of years of unstable life and work circumstances made it difficult to believe I would ever be in the right time and space to stop taking medication. I never really stabilized after that nine months of on-off withdrawal.

Finally, I was in secure employment, feeling brave and happy enough to ditch the drugs. I spent a year weaning off from 75mg, to 37.5, to 25 and then 12.5 to 0mg. Even with an unexpected and sudden redundancy in the middle of it, everything was well until I got to 12.5mg. At this point I was working abroad again in a refugee camp, and it was probably the worst of circumstances I could have continued my taper in. But STILL I had no idea about withdrawal, I didn't know how delicately I had to go. My GP had been unhappy with my tapering plan, saying I didn't need the smaller doses because they weren't manufactured, and discouraging me from opening my capsules to get down to the 25mg and 12.5mg doses. I was cautious, so I continued with this taper regime that my GP thought was 'unnecessary'. So on the facts presented to me by my GP, I had no reason to believe the taper was unsafe for me and I continued.

Things started to unravel at 12.5mg, which I thought was shock and secondary trauma of being in a harrowing environment. Delusions and sleep disturbances began at this point. Vivid nightmares, the feeling of doom and being unsafe began to accompany me everywhere, and I had persistent migraines and vertigo. Still, I continued my taper. Why, why, why?

Because I was so completely and utterly ignorant to withdrawal and had a lack of regard for myself and how I was feeling. I also believed everything I was experiencing was a result of my context, and whilst I would now say it was absolutely contributory and my mind had plentiful material to play with, I believe the one wouldn't have existed without the other.

Although I've no doubt I wouldn't have become quite so ill if I'd been in a safer, more stable environment, I also wouldn't have become so ill organically without the chemical harm that came from withdrawal. I finally stopped taking it, jumping from 12.5mg to 0mg, a taper which my doctor had thought was too slow. I don't know what date I stopped, or how soon after I became acutely unwell, but I developed psychosis within days.

Thankfully, I have an astute and caring partner who did everything he could to keep me safe and get me help. I saw my GP twice in this time, during which he asked if I was 'planning to do anything silly' when I disclosed my suicidal ideation, and twice he resolutely refused to refer me to psychiatry when I asked. After some psychotic behavior and hallucinations, my partner made an urgent self-referral for me and I was assessed by the community mental health team the following day. They were less than helpful, and still no one mentioned withdrawal, but I got back on venlafaxine 37.5mg that day and also walked away with diazepam. That put an end to the kindling psychosis. My psychic pain, panic, insomnia and suicidal ideation continued less dramatically for a further six months, during which time my partner was asked to stop calling the community mental health team as they would offer no further support. Eventually I went back onto my original dose of 75mg of Effexor (brand of venlafaxine) just before my 30th birthday and finally stabilized.

It's now been over four years since I went back onto venlafaxine after the psychosis brought on by withdrawal. In this time I've researched and read about antidepressant withdrawal. I've realized my taper was far, far too fast, despite what my doctor said. I've read about and spoken with hundreds of other people who have been clinically harmed by venlafaxine. I've tapered down slowly at 10% tapers from 75mg to 15mg of Venlafaxine, and found myself stuck unable to go any lower due to the extreme withdrawal symptoms and return of suicidal ideation. I've started and quit a professional training, unable to continue because of the withdrawal effects. I've had to work part time in less stressful roles, giving up my career. I've wanted to have a child, and come to find deeply disturbing anecdotal evidence and research studies that point toward antidepressants being very harmful in-utero. I am not only concerned about miscarriages and having ten fingers and ten toes, I'm worried about the lifelong effects of these drugs on the next generation, which we don't yet know about. I'm concerned that if this drug has caused such havoc with my central nervous system, what would it do the developing nervous system of a fetus and what long term effects will that have? I am now not naive enough to imagine there wouldn't be any.

I've felt that everything in my life is on hold because of the trauma these drugs are causing me. I've been desperate to get off venlafaxine as swiftly as possible, so I could begin to think about moving forward with my career and having a family, but found myself stuck at 15mg with debilitating physiological and emotional withdrawal effects if I went any lower. I decided to 'bridge' onto fluoxetine (Prozac), a method advised by Dr. David Healy, and I experienced such migraines and vertigo that I had to take a relatively much higher dose of Prozac to counteract the withdrawal symptoms. Lucky for me, this 'bridge' worked and I was able to ditch the venlafaxine entirely -however I am clearly so sensitized to withdrawal I couldn't get off the Prozac as quickly as the bridging method suggests. The tapering off from 20mg which I've been doing for the past fourteen months has been challenging. The same withdrawal exists for me, but it is more manageable. With each 10% taper I get around two weeks of withdrawal symptoms, often this has verged into suicidal ideation. I've been managing my symptoms with diet, exercise, psychotherapy, holistic therapies and supplements.

I have still received no meaningful or helpful care from my doctor, and no follow-on support from the psychiatrists who saw me in 2016. I'm still waiting for this nightmare to be over, and once it is I will need to wait some more to see if I am truly stable before I embark on any journey to having a child. I wonder why, as a young woman taking antidepressants for the entirety of my twenties, I was never warned about withdrawal or spoken with about the effect antidepressants would have if I became pregnant? I am so grateful I am not one of the tens of women I have spoken to who have become pregnant only to be withdrawn swiftly from their antidepressants due to the risk, their doctors ignorant of the harm of withdrawal. I am fearful that I may be more at risk of post-natal depression and psychosis, and vulnerable to having to accept medication once again. After my experience, I believe it's imperative we achieve informed consent for everyone who is offered antidepressants, to include an awareness of the likelihood of dependence and withdrawal, and for doctors to have a conversation with all women around their reproductive rights. I think it's imperative that every time someone stops an antidepressant and experiences worsening mental health or physiological symptoms, that doctors are well informed enough to recognize withdrawal. To taper them slowly and let them know there will be adverse effects, rather than simply prescribe another drug and put the symptoms down to their mental health condition. I was told that I was experiencing a 'relapse of depression,', which was proof that I need the medication long term, but I never understood how I could relapse to a place I'd never been before. We need withdrawal to be researched and understood so doctors can recognize and treat it effectively. So treatment might empower patients rather than leave them believing they cannot be well without drugs, all the while experiencing unknown harm from those drugs."

—*From direct submission*

"I am suffering from the effects of withdrawing from antidepressants, having taken them for over 20 years. I was originally prescribed these drugs to treat headaches, the drug was venlafaxine.

Over the years, the dosage was increased to 225mg per day. During this period, I was also prescribed another antidepressant, amitriptyline, which I was told also acts as a pain relief for the headaches I was experiencing. At no point was I advised, throughout these 20 years, of the impact of withdrawing or a review of my medication other than to increase the dosage if my symptoms seemed worse. In hindsight and from research, I now believe my symptoms were that of withdrawal rather than the original complaint getting worse.

About 3½ years ago, I started having anxiety issues about my deceased father. My GP arranged for an appointment with a mental health facility to see if they could offer an alternative treatment, as I expressed I wanted to decrease the venlafaxine because I was tired and unable to function some days. After speaking to a clinician at the center, who liaised with a senior consultant, the outcome of this visit was to increase my 225g daily dosage!! My GP suggested a different antidepressant (he thought I had been taking them for too long, which is an understatement) and gave me a timetable to taper off venlafaxine before starting the new drug.

However, the timescales were too drastic and the amount of reduction made me feel very unwell. I was stuttering and lost all ability to function. He also prescribed Valium to cope 'as and when' I needed them. Again with hindsight this practice of poly-drugging makes the impact of withdrawal much worse. I was not advised of any dangers about coming off the drug so quickly and was left with devastating results to my health. I couldn't work and have never been able to resume because of the impact withdrawal has had on my life and family. My husband had to a stay off work to look after me for 5 months because I was very poorly with the withdrawal symptoms but he had to go back to earn money for our mortgage and bills.

Eventually we lost our lovely home because of the impact withdrawal has had. I still suffer after 31 months of stopping the drugs from horrific and debilitating symptoms. I have no life. I battle to survive each day against thoughts of wanting to end this torment but I won't because I know this is withdrawal from a toxic drug and I never suffered from any of these symptoms before taking it. I went to my GP to find relief from the headaches I was experiencing, not for depression. During my nursing career, I was never given any guidance when dispensing antidepressants in terms of its side effects, long term effects or subsequent withdrawal. It's incredible that a prescribed drug, taken by thousands of people, can cause such devastation, yet the health service is oblivious to this widespread suffering and continues to be in denial.

These drugs should never have been prescribed in the first place and should be banned in the future before more lives are taken."

—*From Petition Ref DD*

"I have been supporting and caring for my wife through her severe experience with being prescribed an SSRI antidepressants. The medical profession has failed us in the following ways for over two decades: 1) Unnecessary prescribing of an antidepressant for situational anxiety that could of being resolved through other therapies; 2) Failure to identify serious neurological side effects early on in the treatment. When seizure type side effects were reported to our local doctor, they were dismissed and we were told it was just anxiety, however later on it was diagnosed and confirmed as extrapyramidal side effects from SSRIs. These have developed into debilitating movement disorders; 3) Inadequate knowledge of withdrawal symptoms leading the doctor to think it was the original condition but in fact the drug. The withdrawal symptoms have been far worse than the original problem. This has led to her dose being increased and yet again chronic use as developed.

As a consequence of all of this, my wife's health has deteriorated rapidly over the years. She has gone from a normal functioning person, working and studying to being completely incapacitated. She has always taking care of herself through diet and exercise and does not drink or smoke, but yet a legally prescribed pill has left her this way. This has impacted us financially as I have to work longer hours to make up for the loss of income. Also the time taking from work to care for her.

Emotionally, this has been devastating, to watch someone suffer at the hands of these drugs is truly heartbreaking. When the withdrawal and side effects from these drugs are so severe that a person is so incapacitated to the point of not even being able to feed themselves or stand up, you have to ask yourself what an earth are these pills doing to someone's brain. Are they the new age lobotomy? Do doctors even know the mechanism of how these drug works? Mr. Marsh, who is now one of Britain's most eminent neurosurgeons, says lobotomies was simply bad science. "It reflected very bad medicine, bad science, because it was clear the patients who were subjected to this procedure were never followed up properly. If you saw the patient after the operation they'd seem alright, they'd walk and talk and say thank you doctor," he observes. The fact they were totally ruined as social human beings probably didn't count.

So are we not just replacing surgical instruments for potent chemicals? I ask again, is prescribing these drugs just a new age lobotomy? It is clear that prescribing antidepressants will continue as the medical profession is so greatly influenced by the pharmaceutical companies. They seem to justify this prescribing by still claiming that it is necessary due to a chemical imbalance in the brain, even though there is no evidence to prove this theory. The fact that my wife goes to the doctor to get her script filled and is never asked how she is on the drug, any side effects occurring etc. just shows there is no interest or concern in getting her to discontinue the drug and highlights the need for it to be used long term. This is certainly not just the case with just a handful of GPs, it is with a majority of them over the years. We have moved house and still with the change of doctors we get the same response. Again, why are these doctors so uneducated about these drugs?

After going on online support forums with my wife, we found she was not the only one being severely affected by these drugs and that many people have similar stories. I certainly don't feel like she has just fallen through the cracks and is a rare case, she is just one of many who are suffering in silence. If the medical profession still insist on prescribing these demon drugs, there should be at least stricter guidelines for the reason for prescribing and certainly emphasis on discontinuing the drug after a certain time. Apart from profiting from money, I will never understand why anyone would want to chemically mess with the delicate neurotransmitters in someone's brain. The fact that I learnt that these drugs were only trialed for six weeks was pretty scary, so what are these drugs actually doing long term? Again, are we heading into lobotomy territory?

It was once considered that Valium could not cause addiction and withdrawal; to me it just sounds like history is repeating itself. Pharmaceutical companies must be laughing all the way to the bank because everyone is so fooled into their great business plan. Let's use the doctors as uneducated pawns to prescribe the drugs and get people dependent because they can't discontinue. It appears that when any problem arises with these drugs no one seems to want to investigate or take responsibility for it. They either put the blame back on the patient or blame is passed in a circle to the doctor, the FDA, back to the patient again but never ever THE DRUGS. There needs to be a thorough investigation into the prescribing and monitoring of all psychiatric drugs in the medical profession. In addition, informed consent of exactly how the drug is supposedly helping their condition, the side effects and risks involved.

Another area that needs to be addressed is the lack of knowledge about withdrawal. Doctors seem to think that 4–6 weeks is a sufficient time to discontinue psychiatric drugs; this is the equivalent to abruptly stopping or going cold turkey, particularly for someone who has been on the drugs for many years. Laurie Oakley's Pharmaceutical Rape series on Dr. David Healy's website states exactly what's happening. We have the cast of characters: the violators (marketers, approval of medicine etc.); the accomplices (medical professionals, prescribers); and the victims (people who experience, physical, emotional and mental suffering from these drugs without given consent of the dangers of these drugs). As with sexual rape, the victims of pharmaceutical violation are everywhere, walking among us unrecognized. Many may not even connect what they experience to their medications. This is a violation involving physical, emotional, mental, social, and spiritual damage at the hands of those holding power over medicines, who deny any wrongdoing and remain free to do the same to others".

—From Petition Ref AAAAAA

"I would like to share my story, in order to highlight the harm that I believe is caused by SSRI and SNRI antidepressants. In 2008, I suffered the horrendous experience of a depressive psychosis. It was diagnosed by psychiatry as 'postnatal psychosis'. I now have a strong suspicion that my psychosis was caused, or at least exacerbated, by SSRIs.

My first daughter was born in April 2008. I took citalopram at a steady dose for about 2 years prior to the birth and throughout my pregnancy. In the days after she was born, I read that sertraline was the safest SSRI to take while breastfeeding. I asked the GP about it and she changed me from citalopram to sertraline. In the following weeks I became very depressed. I was changed back to citalopram and the dose was fairly rapidly increased.

In the weeks following this, I became suicidally depressed and developed a florid depressive psychosis. I made several suicide attempts and started to think I had a duty to kill my baby to release her from the awful suffering that the world would cause her. Fortunately for us all, before I acted on those thoughts, I was sectioned. I continued on citalopram and olanzapine was added. I did not respond quickly to the meds so was given ECT. I had a fairly rapid improvement following ECT and was allowed home. However, after a few months my depressive psychosis returned. I was changed to venlafaxine and quetiapine and after 3 months the depressive psychosis lifted and I remained well until two years after the birth of my second daughter in 2012. I was advised to take quetiapine for some months after this birth.

I remained well for two years; however, following a period of stress and no longer on quetiapine, I had another episode of depressive psychosis. I remained on venlafaxine but this time quetiapine was not effective. My antipsychotic was changed to amisulpride and after 3 months I recovered. I have remained on a low dose of amisulpride and have not experienced psychosis since then. I appreciate that it is very difficult to prove, but I now wonder about the possibility that I have a sensitivity to SSRIs/SNRIs and that my episodes of psychosis were actually caused by citalopram/venlafaxine and that the psychosis was only subdued by the addition of an antipsychotic. I was told on a number of occasions by the psychiatry team that my illness was 'atypical.' I do not remember any of the psychiatry team ever mentioning the possibility that my psychosis may have been caused/exacerbated by SSRIs—it was always attributed to an underlying illness, be it 'postnatal psychosis' or 'psychotic depression.' This has led me to wonder how many other cases of psychosis may be influenced by these drugs, which is why I want to highlight the issue. If psychiatry is not considering this possibility, this potential cause will not be being reported and it could be going unnoticed, meaning it is possible that, like me, some people are advised to continue on the drugs that precipitated their psychosis in the first place, with further treatments being added to counteract the negative effects of the SSRI/SNRI.

I would also like to highlight the problems I have had attempting to withdraw from venlafaxine. In discussion with my psychiatrist, I decided to come off venlafaxine in 2015, having been well for over two years. My psychiatrist recommended a taper which I now believe was way too fast -over several weeks. The withdrawal during those weeks was a truly awful experience. For the whole period of withdrawal and several weeks afterwards, I felt like I had a severe bout of the flu and a terrible hangover. I had electric shock sensations in my head. It felt as if my brain was being constantly irritated by a chemical. I felt agitated and intensely irritable. I felt an intense burning sensation in my head, spine and esophagus. My body ached all over. I had abdominal pain. I lost my senses of taste and smell. Then approximately three months after stopping venlafaxine, I became depressed. I completely lost my appetite and felt a physical sensation of my body and mind being an empty shell, unlike anything I had ever experienced. I was admitted to a psychiatric unit. My bowel stopped working. I was put back on venlafaxine and after approximately four months I fairly suddenly started to feel better again. The physical symptoms disappeared. The psychiatry team were convinced the whole episode was caused by my underlying illness—'psychotic depression,' because my depression could not be controlled without venlafaxine. However, I always suspected that what I experienced was a very bad case of withdrawal from venlafaxine.

Recently I decided I would like to try to withdraw from venlafaxine again, but this time much, much more slowly. I found a Facebook group dedicated to venlafaxine withdrawal. It has approximately 3800 members. Time and time again people report that they were not warned about the difficulties that many people have withdrawing from venlafaxine—indeed most medical professionals seem completely unaware of the problem that so many of us experience. The recommended taper advised in the group is a maximum of 10% of the dose at a time, with a hold of at least 30 days or until all withdrawal symptoms have resolved, before tapering again. For many of us, particularly those of us who have been taking it for a number of years, it would seem that to have the best chance of getting off venlafaxine and staying well we must reduce the dose very gradually over years. There are members of the group who, like me, came off much more quickly on the advice of their psychiatrist/GP, did not reinstate the drug quickly enough and who have suffered a protracted withdrawal over years, with a whole host of symptoms.

I can't help but feel that if there could be a much greater understanding of antidepressant withdrawal amongst medical professionals, including revised guidelines for withdrawal in the community, then more of us would receive the support we need to come off venlafaxine and other psychiatric drugs, rather than suffering intense withdrawal symptoms and being told that they are nothing to do with withdrawal but are the return of our original illness. I find it very interesting in relation to my suspicion that I experienced SSRI induced psychosis that, since reducing my venlafaxine dose from 150mg to 100mg, my thoughts seem less distorted and obsessive, I have less anxiety, my thinking is much clearer, I have more energy and I am much less drowsy."

—*From Petition Ref BBBBBBBB*

"In 2011, my doctor diagnosed me with mild depression and fibromyalgia pain, and against my better judgment, I started taking Ciprelex. I was told it was the new latest antidepressant, and was told there would be no withdrawals when coming off them. (I realize now my doctor was just repeating what the drug rep told him, and what literature he had read from the drug company. I'm sure he thought this was a new safer drug to use for treating depression and fibromyalgia pain.)

Shortly after taking Ciprelex, I noticed electrical shocks, and a burning sensation going through my brain and body (to the point I was afraid to drive or operate machinery). I talked to my doctor and was told this was my body getting used to the chemical change in my body, and only a few experience this. I felt it wasn't really helping me and my dose was increased from 10mg to 20mg a day. This drug basically made me into a functioning zombie; shortly after taking this drug, I found I could no longer function and do my job as a consultant/ mechanical engineer in the oil fields (17 years). I used to be very good at organizing, producing reports, troubleshooting, and staying calm in difficult situations, doing math in my head.

My life turned into a nightmare, I started having very violent and gory dreams (which was very unusual for me) and started having suicidal thoughts (again, unusual for me). I was having trouble with my eyesight shortly after going on this drug, saw an optometrist, and was told it was my age was catching up to me, but could not explain why I developed 'night blindness.' (Having read reports, I am now finding out a lot of people on these drugs have developed 'night blindness' and other eye problems.) For me, it was to the point where I would not drive at night, and still won't. Some of the littlest daily problems can get me overwhelmed very easily.

The list of side effects from this drug for me was very severe and long. The scary thing about it is I didn't realize or understand that it was the drug doing this to me. I felt I was on the outside looking in. Due to my behavior I could not hold down jobs, did not get along with other coworkers, was actually let go from a job (for the first time in my life) after being a longtime employee at other jobs, always getting along with everyone. I became a recluse, and lost interest in a lot of daily life activities; reading, playing music. I had to shut down a part-time photography and custom picture framing business (which was my passion). I was severely depressed, suicidal, physically sick, suffered severe episodes of anxiety (which was unusual for me). I had severe 'brain fog,' insomnia, etc. I felt I had spiritually died inside, and felt I was dying physically to the point that I purchased a body bag. My 'distorted' thinking being if I died, or committed suicide, I didn't want to leave a mess for others to deal with; this way, it would be contained.

After an unusual night of clarity, I was reflecting on my life and how terrible it had gotten, I realized it started, or had changed since taking Ciprelex (2.5 years). I knew I had to get off of it. I talked to my doctor and told him I wanted to get off Ciprelex, and he agreed and we started slowly weaning off the dosage. This turned into another nightmare all in itself (it was just horrible) as withdrawal was very severe. The doctor and pharmacist kept telling me it was just my body getting used to the chemical change in my body, and it would only last 6 weeks (again both repeating what the drug literature, and drug reps had told them). I had to go back on a higher dose of Ciprelex , and try a slower weaning off which took 6 months, still with very severe side effects. (This sounds like withdrawal to me, even though the drug companies said there would be no withdrawal).

I have now been off Ciprelex for six years, and am still dealing with the side effects, and possible brain damage. I ended up selling just about everything I owned, and moved to live with family (who are still having difficulty in understanding what the hell happened to me). I have seen other doctors, psychologists who say no, it's not the Ciprelex, as it will only stay in the body for 6 weeks. (When I hear this, I know they have been indoctrinated by the pharmaceutical companies, as most doctors do not have a clue what these drugs are capable of.) I still have not been able to get back to work or function normally. Even after six years of being off Ciprelex, I still get electrical shocks and brain zaps (as a lot of people try to describe them), and I never had these effects until I started taking Ciprelex. There is severe memory loss from the past five years, as many others have experienced also. And just to list a few more side effects, dysphoria, akathisia, PTSD, anhedonia; I have been in and out of emergency rooms, but most doctors offer very little help, and do not know how to deal with this, a lot of time making the situation life threating.

I could go on and on, as this is just a little snapshot of what I, and many others are going through, and the hell they are dealing with. We are not going crazy we just have been poisoned, and trying to find out if the brain damage is permanent, or temporary?

I understand why people go back on these drugs after trying to get off them. It's horrible. I have since found a new doctor who is aware of what's going on with these drugs. These drugs can stay in your system for a very long time as I, and others are finding out (not the six-week period like we were told by the drug companies) and are proving to be very damaging to the brain. In desperation when coming off Ciprelex, I went and saw an addiction counselor, who told me antidepressants are becoming a 'huge' problem for them.

Yes, they are very, very addictive and very damaging drugs. Having researched and talking with many others, I am finding I am not an isolated and unusual case. Just one of the sites I'm a member of on Facebook (and there are many of them), which includes almost 4000 people from all over (again, this is just from ONE site) are experiencing the same problems I am, in one form or another, from taking these drugs. This information needs to get out to more people. There are thousands suffering in silence, and they're not gone, or going crazy, they have been poisoned! I have lost everything that was dear to me, my career, marriage, my house, my music, my passions, my spirituality, my life savings. I could write more, but I think you get part of the picture."

—From Petition Ref FF

"Over the past 12 years, I have been existing in an Orwellian/Kafkaesque nightmare of psychiatric drugs, psychiatrists and hospitals. It started when I was put on the antidepressant Cipralex in 2005 after a prolonged period of stress which culminated in me being in London on the day of the 7/7 terrorist attacks. Despite only taking a couple of tablets, I developed what I now know is a condition called akathisia—an intense state of agitation. I stopped taking the tablets immediately, but after a month of severe anxiety, being unable to eat or sleep, I was admitted to a private psychiatric hospital where they prescribed me the antipsychotic olanzapine off label (i.e. not approved for that use). Two days later, I was suicidal.

I had never ever been suicidal before. Over the next 10 years I tried numerous times to kill myself: overdoses, attempted drowning, strangulation, trying to throw myself under a train, you name it. Over the next 10 years, I saw nine further psychiatrists and in total I was put on 15 different drugs. They told me I had severe depressive disorder. I was anxious, depressed, emotionally blunted, agoraphobic as well as suicidal. Not one of these so called 'medical experts' recognized that I was having a catastrophic reaction to the drugs. They just kept chopping and changing the drugs, upping and lowering the doses, starting and stopping at the drop of a hat. I was even offered electroconvulsive therapy, which I declined. I didn't fancy having my brain fried.

During 2017, I spent 10 months withdrawing from the final two drugs venlafaxine and mirtazapine. This combination has a nickname—'California Rocket Fuel.' You can imagine what that was doing to my poor nervous system. At times I felt so ill I thought I was going to die. Sometimes I have had to spend days on end in bed. Early last year, my blood pressure was skyrocketing and I had to call the paramedics out twice. I finished my last dose just before Christmas. Since then I have been suffering from severe insomnia, skin rashes, gastrointestinal problems and burning/aching sensations over the whole of my body. I have no idea when and if this will ever go away. I have also been trying to lose some of the 50+ lbs. in weight that I put on due to these drugs. I am quite likely to end up with type 1 insulin dependent diabetes after 10 years on olanzapine, as it is one of the major effects of this drug.

I have lost my home, my kids, my relationships, my physical health and I am completely traumatized. At one point a year ago I was virtually destitute: homeless, broke, ill and terrified. I had even been on the receiving end of mental abuse by my own family who just do not seem to understand. I nearly got sectioned when a psychiatrist turned up where I was staying, accompanied by two henchmen who threatened to put me in hospital, back on olanzapine. I was absolutely terrified.

Once you are in the mental health system, it is very hard to get out of it. I have managed it, but even then they have damned me further by giving me another totally subjective label of schizo-affective disorder. They have tried to put me on a further antipsychotic, quetiapine which I have refused to take. So what have these wonderful drugs done for me? Basically they have totally and utterly destroyed my life. Am I angry? No, I am absolutely incandescent with rage. If you look at the statistics produced by The Samaritans, you will find that despite skyrocketing rates of antidepressant prescribing, suicide rates across the UK have changed little over the past 30 years. An article on the website AntiDepAware recently quoted NHS statistics from a Dundee Evening Telegraph article which reported that between 2009 and 2015, 147 people took their own lives in Dundee. In 2016, numbers reached 37—the highest annual figure for 21 years. More than 87% of these people were apparently taking antidepressant medication. Rather makes a mockery of the idea that these drugs save lives, doesn't it?"

—From Petition Ref JJJJJJJ

"I write my story only in hope that I can save people from ever getting on an antidepressant and/or benzodiazepine. I am a married 45 year old businesswoman with two beautiful children who are 13 and 15 years old. I have my Bachelor of Science degree in Human Services and currently work as an Account Executive. Most recently, I was on Lexapro for 12 years. I actually think I had been on something else when I was pregnant, but I honestly cannot remember due to the short-term memory loss these drugs have caused.

I was originally prescribed Lexapro for an eating disorder (bulimia) and well as OCD tendencies. The Lexapro gave me insomnia so the doctor also put me on a sleeping pill called Lunesta. When I switched over health insurances to Kaiser, the doctor told me they do not cover Lunesta as it is too addicting and asked that I try another 'sleeping pill' called Klonopin. Little did I know Klonopin is worse than Xanax and that it was extremely addicting. I was taking 2mg of Klonopin for over 2 years. I also started gaining weight so the doctor also put me on another pill called phentermine. I was on two doses of 37.5mg of phentermine daily for over six years.

Meanwhile, I have never done drugs my whole life nor barely even drink alcohol. When I found out all these drugs were addicting, I got nervous so I started lowering my dose of all the pills over a 10-week period (which I now know was way too fast). By June 1st, 2016, I was off all the drugs. My initial withdrawals were not so bad…then bam came the third month and ALL hell broke loose! I literally had almost every withdrawal symptom possible and they only got worse as the days went on. I was like a complete vegetable; I couldn't see well, hear well, I was confused, had a hard time comprehending simple things, felt out of my body, racing thoughts, crying spells, mood swings, sweats, cold chills, flu-like symptoms, nightmares, felt depersonalized, dizzy, disoriented, diarrhea every day, no appetite, sensitive to light, losing my hair…and the list goes on and on. I literally felt like I was living in hell on earth.

As the days turned into weeks then months, things only got worse. I ended up with so much anxiety and depression like I have never experienced before. Then the insomnia kicked in so bad I ended up not sleeping for three straight weeks which made me manic. I was pacing around my house like a crazy woman and I couldn't even sit still. My heart was pounding out of my chest and I literally felt like I had become completely mentally ill. By the sixth month, I became extremely suicidal and tried to take my life by hanging myself. I had/have no recollection of this event as I literally became that mentally ill. I was placed on a 5150 and put in a mental ward for 10 days. It was literally the worst experience of my life.

In the hospital, they tried to drug me up again. I was given Luvox, Zyprexa (which I refused to take) and Xanax five times per day. The doctor would not even listen to my story nor lend me five minutes of his time. In the hospital, I was still completely out of it and couldn't even sleep. I felt like a complete zombie. After I was released, I was forced to move in with my 75 year old mother for a month as I couldn't even care for myself nor let my children see me in the condition I was in. I then began to have an allergic reaction to the Luvox, so I slowly cross tapered over to 10mg of Prozac and got back on a low dose of Klonopin.

As of today, I am only on 10mg of Prozac and thankfully off the Klonopin and phentermine! I've been off the Lexapro and phentermine for 19 months now and the Klonopin for 8 months but am still feeling weird. It's been 14 months since I was hospitalized and although I am much better, I still don't feel completely like myself. I am back to work full-time but I'm not sure if I'm still going through withdrawals from all the previous meds or if it's side effects from the Prozac. As of today, I am still losing my hair and have to wear a wig full time because of all the hair loss. I was recently diagnosed with Androgenic Alopecia related to this situation. My memory and vision are still horrible, but thankfully are slowly starting to get better. I still have trouble sleeping and am dizzy at times as well.

I feel flat, with no happiness or joy. I never want to do things and nothing really bothers me now. I am forcing myself to get out of the house and do things with my family and friends. Since this nightmare of an experience happened, this is all I think about. I absolutely hate that I'm still on this poison, but honestly believe the only reason I got better was because I went back on a medication. I honestly believe I would still be sick/mentally ill had I stayed off everything and that is what's so traumatizing. I am scared to death to start my taper from Prozac in fear of going through withdrawals again. My plan is to start a slow three-year taper in another four months or so. If I successfully complete it, I will definitely be making my story public in hopes to educate people on these poisons!"

—*From Petition Ref GGGGG*

CONCLUSION

TAKING OR NOT taking antidepressants is an individual's choice. Being informed about the evidence-based risks and benefits of antidepressants is an individual's right. Encouraging each other to question and learn about our options for treatment is fundamental if we are to change the way we think about how we treat our "mental health". We need to wake up to the fact the current way we choose to cope with the more difficult times in our lives is guided by neither evidence-based science nor best practice.

This book has not been about politics or "Big Pharma bashing" it has been about helping us make informed choices about antidepressants and changing how we think about and talk about coping with the difficult times in our lives.

Dainus Pūras believes we need to address the social determinants of mental health and looks at inequalities in daily life and social exclusion as major problems. "The urgent need for a shift in approach should prioritize policy innovation at the population level, targeting social determinants and abandon the predominant medical model that seeks to cure individuals by targeting 'disorders'. The crisis in mental health should be managed not as a crisis of individual conditions, but as a crisis of social obstacles which hinders individual rights. Mental health policies should address the 'power imbalance' rather than the chemical imbalance."[240]

This book has revealed some of the obstacles hindering our individual rights to safe and effective treatment, while acknowledging the wider context. Reforms in mental health laws, policies, and practices are urgently needed as we become increasingly all too aware of the unquantifiable "crisis of individual conditions" which needs to urgently be addressed.

The power imbalance of our mental health system has left us open to our inabilities to cope with life being commercially and politically exploited. The pharmaceutical industry and psychiatry have capitalized on the fact we believe and accept antidepressants and other medications are a safe and effective answer to our problems. It has somehow become acceptable for governments to fail to acknowledge and address the social determinants affecting our lives. They have made us believe it is our fault and not theirs.

This biomedical approach to mental health, that mental disorders are brain diseases and that any medication-based treatment targets the abnormalities involved in the brain, has dominated the American Health Care system for over thirty years, since the introduction Prozac. The most powerful voices such as the National Alliance on Mental Illness (NAMI) and Mental Health America (MHA) promote mental health as being just like physical health, diseases and illness. The language is that of psychiatry with the tone of the smiling assassin. The MHA tag #B4Stage4, is a comparison to cancer or other physical disease treatment. There is an emphasis to "Get Screened" and "Identify the underlying illness."[241]

The National Alliance on Mental Illness (NAMI) proudly declares it receives generous support from numerous partners including Pfizer, Teva, Bristol Myers Squibb, Janssen, Eli Lilly and Lundbeck. It openly collaborates with the American Psychiatric Association. In 2009, the New York Times revealed, "A majority of the donations made to the National Alliance on Mental Illness, one of the nation's most influential disease advocacy groups, have come from drug makers in recent years, according to Congressional investigators." "Drug makers are natural allies in these pursuits since cures may come out of corporate laboratories and the industry's money can help finance public service campaigns and fund-raising dinners. But industry critics have long derided some patient organizations as little more than front groups devoted to lobbying on issues that affect industry profits, and few have come under more scrutiny for industry ties than the mental health alliance."[242]

It all adds up to the powerful promotion of a medical model of mental health disguised as advocacy. They subtly communicate mental disorders are brain diseases and the model they use tells us we need drugs to target our brain abnormalities and to reverse an underlying disease. In her article in the Journal of Bioethical Inquiry, Sharon Batt, a bioethicist from Dalhousie University, Canada, sums up the situation: "Accepting industry money would result in vulnerable patients being susceptible to the parroting of certain marketing messages that distorted scientific evidence, with the potential to cause needless suffering, misplaced hope, premature deaths, and misspent funds."[243]

This bombardment of mental health messages isn't keeping us healthy. It is being strategically used by the powerful to avoid responsibility. It enables governments to shy away from dealing with the social determinants of our stress, anxiety and unhappiness. We live with poverty, loneliness, homelessness, abuse, unemployment and the many other social and environmental factors causing our distress, but we are told it is all about our "mental health". They tell us the problem is "our" mental health and "we" need to fix it. It is our mental health that is our problem, our illness or condition. It is a clever avoidance strategy to keep our attention away from the investments needed in society to provide the resources to enable us to live happy and healthy lives. We need psychosocial solutions, and we need to realize it is life that is our problem and not the chemicals in our brain. Our social problems have in turn conveniently become medical ones and it makes life easier and more profitable for those at the top.

The mental health monster, born with Prozac in the late 1980s, is an invasive creature trampling every aspect of society in the developed world with no intention of stopping there. New markets are in sight and the untreated and seemingly neglected nations will soon be the focus for the continuing growth of pharmaceutical psychotropic interventions. The fastest growing market, according to the Global Antidepressants Market research report 2019[244], is Asia Pacific. "Asia Pacific is the fastest growing region for antidepressants and portrays huge potential for growth in the future due to an increasing prevalence of psychiatric disorders and rapid economic growth in this region." The most naturally resilient nations in the world are the next antidepressant target market.

The COVID-19 pandemic has created somewhat hysterical fear and talk of worldwide "mental illness." Whilst some speak of millions suffering PTSD or Depressive Disorders, others such as Dr. Lucy Johnstone have taken a somewhat more realistic view of our situation. "Surviving the pandemic, as most of us will, is only the start of it. However, we must not be tempted back into a medical narrative, even though the aftermath will probably be as bad, if not worse. Healthcare staff may be deeply shaken by the suffering they saw, but we don't have to call it an outbreak of 'PTSD'. People who have lost their jobs are likely to feel desperate, but we don't have to describe this as 'clinical depression' and prescribe drugs for it. The economic recession that will follow the pandemic may lead to as many suicides as austerity measures did, but we don't have to say that 'mental illness' caused these deaths. The drug companies must be rubbing their hands at the prospect of all these new customers. We can come out of this crisis in a better state than before by staying connected with our feelings and the urgent threats that have led to them and taking collective action to deal with the root causes."[245]

At a time when there is talk of a mental health epidemic, there has never been a more appropriate time to question the medicalizing of our emotional distress. Mental illness is not a disease and therefore not really an epidemic... it never was and never will be, but unless we challenge the current mental health narrative, unless we educate ourselves and learn about the powerful drugs we take, we will see more suffering, illness and deaths.[246] There has perhaps never been a better time for change.

Dainius Pūras talks of existing alternatives to our current mental health system and the quiet revolution he sees happening: "Such alternative practices with transformative potential have been in existence for decades, with many shown to be effective. They take many shapes and forms, from the commendable global work of WHO with its Quality Rights initiative on improving the quality of mental health care and services, to systems-level community health reforms in Brazil and Italy, to highly localized innovations in different resource settings around the world, such as Soteria House, Open Dialogue, peer-respite centers, medication-free wards. A quiet revolution has been occurring in neighborhoods and communities worldwide. At the root of these alternatives is a deep commitment to human rights, dignity and non-coercive practices, all of which remain an elusive challenge in traditional mental health systems too heavily reliant on a biomedical paradigm."[247]

There is growing awareness of the need for that "paradigm shift in mental health" but as Dainius Pūras states, "What that shift looks like in practice is a matter of much debate." Whilst governments around the world debate, medics remain willfully blind and charities secure their funding, the change has to start with us as individuals, as advocates and as informed patients. The fact that we know a doctor's appointment is often the start of a lifelong journey as a psychiatric patient with a stigmatizing lifelong condition and dependence on psychiatric medication means the shift starts by us questioning the overuse of antidepressants and looking at alternative ways to support and care for each other. It starts by becoming more knowledgeable, reclaiming some control and power over our own healthcare and by taking responsibility to educate ourselves to the best of our ability. It starts by understanding antidepressants are not the easy and quick fix their makers and doctors say they are. It starts with the acceptance we might be doing more harm than good by defining ourselves using mental health labels and diagnoses. Life is difficult and we have all probably faced some degree of trauma, stress and unhappiness in our life. We all have unmet needs or times when life becomes too challenging and it is time to accept it is mostly about social causes and not biological ones.

Prescribed drugs associated with dependence and withdrawal have been described as "a significant public health issue, one that is central to doctors' clinical role, and one that the medical profession has a clear responsibility to help address."[248] This is true throughout the developed world. The following actions and considerations are amongst those needed to prevent more overprescribing, harm and dependence.

Prescribing guidelines must be adhered to and antidepressants should not be first-line treatment. Doctors should recommend watchful waiting where appropriate. If we choose to take antidepressants, we should be advised to take them for the shortest time possible and long-term antidepressant use should be discouraged. We should be reviewed frequently. Off-label prescribing of antidepressants should be avoided where possible.

We need informed consent for antidepressant treatment. This means we understand why, based on our diagnosis, the treatment is being offered and we are aware of the benefits and risks. Only then should we agree to the treatment. Informed consent is our medical right.

There is a need for better education of medical professionals about the dangers of antidepressants including the potential for dependence. We urgently need evidence-based withdrawal protocols. The developed world must address the issue of antidepressant deprescribing and withdrawal as a matter of urgency. The FDA and APA need to update guidelines on antidepressant withdrawal.

Prescribing antidepressants to children and young people should be questioned. Governments, medics and other mental health organizations need to recognize antidepressant-induced suicide as a leading cause, particularly amongst the young. Everyone must learn about akathisia.

We urgently need support services for those harmed by or dependent on antidepressants. There is currently little support available for those of us withdrawing from antidepressants. The medical profession must stop misdiagnosing withdrawal as relapse and unnecessarily increasing medications. We need to question why we need to turn to unregulated peer-led services for help.

We need investment in psychosocial interventions as first-line treatment, and these should be available at a community level to everyone who is experiencing mental health issues. We need to question whether or not our human needs can really be met by psychotropic drugs.

The FDA advises, "Be an active member of your health care team. By taking time to learn about the possible side effects of a drug and working with your health care provider and pharmacist, you will be better prepared to reduce your chance of experiencing a side effect or coping with any side effect that you may experience."[249] This is very good advice, but we need to be more than an active member of our healthcare team. We need to become informed, educated and we must share our knowledge if we are to reduce the role and impact antidepressants have on our lives and society.

As governments and the medical profession continue to underestimate and ignore the problem, we find ourselves in a situation where, for the current time at least, it is down to the power of patient experience and those of us willing to question the status quo to make change happen. It is suggested we start to think about "what is happening with you?" rather than "what is wrong with you?" It is a good question to ask as it often highlights the true sources of our distress. It is a simple question that could prevent us becoming part of the medicalized mental health system and taking unnecessary medication. Whatever our age, whatever adverse experiences or trauma we might have encountered in our life, we all have a right to reach our full potential and thrive. We all have a right to live a label free and unmedicated life if that is what we choose. We all have a right to question if doctor always knows best when it comes to the "wicked" problem of antidepressants.

THE RESOURCE GUIDE
GENERAL DRUG INFORMATION

SELECTIVE SEROTONIN REUPTAKE INHIBITORS (SSRIs)	
GENERICS	**BRAND NAMES***
Citalopram	Celexa, Cipramil
Escitalopram	Cipralex, Lexapro
Fluoxetine	Prozac, Sarafem
Fluvoxamine	Luvox, Faverin
Paroxetine	Paxil, Seroxat
Sertraline	Zoloft, Lustral

SEROTONIN NOREPINEPHRINE REUPTAKE INHIBITORS (SNRIs)	
GENERICS	**BRAND NAMES***
Desvenlafaxine	Pristiq
Duloxetine	Cymbalta
Levomilnacipran	Fetzima
Milnacipran	Ixel, Savella
Venlafaxine	Effexor
**These drugs have many different brand names throughout the world. Medications might be available in tablet, capsule, or liquid form.*	

Antidepressant	Approximate Half-Life (Hours)
Citalopram	36
Desvenlafaxine	11
Duloxetine	30
Escitalopram	8–17
Fluoxetine	96–144
Fluvoxamine	24
Levomilnacipran	12
Milnacipran	8
Paroxetine	17–22
Sertraline	22–36
Venlafaxine	4–7
Medications might be available in tablet, capsule, or liquid form.	

Where can you go to learn more about prescription drugs and over-the-counter medicines, including side effects, dosage, special precautions, interactions etc.?

- www.medlineplus.gov
- www.drugs.com
- www.pimsplus.org
- www.fda.gov/drugs/resources-you-drugs/drug-information-consumers
- www.medicinenet.com
- www.dailymed.nlm.nih.gov
- www.rxisk.org

USEFUL RESOURCES

Inner Compass Initiative/The Withdrawal Project/Connect

www.theinnercompass.org
Inner Compass Initiative, The Withdrawal Project, ICI Connect, and TWP Connect are web-based online information-sharing and connecting platforms which seek to provide opportunities for likeminded people to find each other, and to facilitate the sharing of information that improves the general public's understanding of psychiatric drug withdrawal and of "mental health" diagnoses and treatments generally. Any and all information, materials, and content posted on the Website is provided for general educational and informational purposes only. Unless expressly stated otherwise, the authors, bloggers, and/or editors of the Website are laypeople who have direct personal experience taking, reducing, or tapering off psychiatric medication and/or supporting someone else who has taken, reduced, or tapered off psychiatric medication.

The Withdrawal Project is an information resource designed to help people empower themselves to make more meaningfully informed choices—aligned with their personal desires and needs—regarding taking, reducing, and coming off psychiatric drugs. TWP's website includes a free, comprehensive, self-directed Companion Guide to Psychiatric Drug Withdrawal aimed at helping people learn and make decisions about the most risk-minimizing ways to prepare for tapering off and more responsibly taper off antidepressants, benzodiazepines, stimulants, antipsychotics, mood stabilizers, Z-drugs and other psychiatric drugs, along with coping techniques for dealing with common withdrawal symptoms.

ICI Connect

ICI Connect is a simple, free online platform that is designed to help people who are asking questions or thinking critically about the mental health system find and connect with each other in person. After creating basic profiles, members can search by location and/or interest for other members who live nearby in order to connect, share information, spark new friendships or collaborations, provide mutual support or advocacy, organize public learning events or groups, set up crisis networks, or begin to build grassroots community alternatives to the mental health system. Our members are generally people who've experienced or witnessed some of the misleading, coercive or harmful aspects of our current mental health system—we're part of a rapidly growing segment of society that has become passionate about developing alternative approaches and building more mutually supportive and socially just communities beyond the mental health system.

Surviving Antidepressants

www.survivingantidepressants.org

SurvivingAntidepressants.org is a site for peer support, documentation, and education regarding tapering and withdrawal syndrome from psychiatric drugs, including antidepressants.

Withdrawal syndrome may occur after you stop taking a psychiatric medication and can last weeks, months, or years. While some people may be able to quickly stop taking these medications without serious symptoms, severe withdrawal syndrome can happen to anyone.

Tapering off the medication is the only known way to reduce the risk of withdrawal syndrome. Don't risk the integrity of your nervous system; if not in an emergency, do not suddenly stop taking any psychiatric medication.

Harm Reduction Guide to Coming Off Psychiatric Drugs /Will Hall

willhall.net
www.freedom-center.org
The Fireweed Collective/Icarus Project and Freedom Center's 52-page illustrated guide gathers the best information and most valuable lessons from more than a decade of peer support community mutual aid. This free guide is used internationally by individuals, families, professionals, and organizations, and is available in more than 14 translations.

RxISK

www.rxisk.org
RxISK is a free, independent drug safety website to help you weigh the benefits of any medication against its potential dangers. In its Antidepressant Guide, it includes information about side effects of antidepressants, stopping antidepressants, notes on antidepressant withdrawal to take to your therapist, and Post-SSRI Sexual Dysfunction (PSSD).

Psychiatric Drug Facts with Dr. Peter Breggin MD

www.breggin.com
Dr. Peter Breggin's Antidepressant Drug Resource & Information Center For Prescribers, Scientists, Professionals, Patients and their Families.

Mad in America

www.madinamerica.com
Mad in America's mission is to serve as a catalyst for rethinking psychiatric care in the United States (and abroad). We believe that the current drug-based paradigm of care has failed our society, and that scientific research, as well as the lived experience of those who have been diagnosed with a psychiatric disorder, calls for profound change.

MIA's withdrawal pages are meant to provide resources, research findings, and personal stories relevant to making informed choices about withdrawing from psychiatric drugs. In addition to the general information on this page, there are links to withdrawal information.

Mad in the UK

www.madintheuk.com

MITUK's mission is to serve as a catalyst for fundamentally re-thinking theory and practice in the field of mental health in the UK, and promoting positive change. We believe that the current diagnostically-based paradigm of care has comprehensively failed, and that the future lies in non-medical alternatives which explicitly acknowledge the causal role of social and relational conflicts, abuses, adversities and injustices.

The Council for Evidence-based Psychiatry

www.cepuk.org

CEP exists to communicate evidence of the potentially harmful effects of psychiatric drugs to the people and institutions in the UK that can make a difference. The scientific record clearly shows that psychiatric medications, portrayed as safe and effective by areas of the medical profession, often lead to worse outcomes for many patients, particularly when taken long term. Our members include psychiatrists, academics, withdrawal support charities and others who are concerned about the prevalence of the 'medical model' and the increasing numbers of prescriptions for psychiatric drugs being given to both adults and children.

Let's Talk Withdrawal

www.letstalkwithdrawal.com

Psychotropic prescription drugs (such as antidepressants, antipsychotics and anxiolytic medications) are often very difficult to stop taking. Users who have come to the end of treatment and wish to stop can suffer debilitating withdrawal symptoms, even when following their doctor's advice. In some cases, these withdrawal symptoms can be so severe that they prevent the user from stopping their medication. This site exists to describe the problem, provide interviews with people who have lived experience and campaign for change.

Medicating Normal

www.medicatingnormal.com
The film acknowledges that psychiatric drugs do help alleviate suffering for a segment of those who take them. However, it is estimated that of the 1 in 5 Americans taking such meds, 30% to 35% are gravely harmed by the very treatment meant to help them. Medicating Normal focuses on the predicament of this group—individuals facing trauma and stress who are drugged needlessly and made sicker as a result. Interviews with experts in the film reveal that significant numbers of these people will get better over time without medication. The website includes information about withdrawal and alternatives.

MIND

www.mind.org.uk/media/8453/coming-off-medication-2021-pdf-version.pdf
Coming Off Psychiatric Drugs. Many people would like to stop their psychiatric medication but coming off can be difficult. This booklet is for people who are thinking about coming off their medication and for friends, family and others who want to support them." Free to download.

Robert Whitaker Books

www.robertwhitakerbooks.com
Robert Whitaker has won numerous awards as a journalist covering medicine and science, including the George Polk Award for Medical Writing and a National Association for Science Writers' Award for best magazine article. In 1998, he co-wrote a series on psychiatric research for the Boston Globe that was a finalist for the Pulitzer Prize for Public Service. Anatomy of an Epidemic won the 2010 Investigative Reporters and Editors book aware for best investigative journalism. He is also

the publisher and founder of Madinamerica.com, a critical psychiatry webzine.

Fiddaman Blog

www.fiddaman.blogspot.com
Author of The Evidence, However, is Clear: The Seroxat Scandal. Researching drug company and regulatory malfeasance for over 16 years. Humanist, humorist.

Akathisia Alliance for Education and Research

www.akathisiaalliance.org
The "Akathisia Alliance for Education and Research" is a nonprofit organization formed by people who have experienced it. Our group includes biochemists, psychologists, nurses, attorneys, business owners, and others who have survived akathisia, suicidality, and devastating personal losses due, in part, to a lack of awareness by medical professionals. We have come together from all walks of life to battle these things we all have in common, so we can help prevent them from happening to others.

MISSD

www.missd.co
MISSD is pleased to now offer Akathisia 101. The free, online one-hour continuing education course is open to all who want to better understand, identify and respond to akathisia. Akathisia 101 is approved by the National Association of Social Workers for 1 continuing education contact hour. Healthcare and crisis teams, patients, therapists, caregivers, doctors, first-responders, drug safety advocates and educators—everyone can benefit from akathisia awareness. Let's make Akathisia a household word."

Bloom in Wellness

www.baylissa.com
Bloom in Wellness is a soothing and uplifting website that was created for anyone wanting a quiet retreat to focus on healing and recovery, and on living one's best life despite challenges. This is a tranquil, private space for you to renew hope and regain your equilibrium if coping with whatever you are facing is difficult and motivation to persevere is waning. It offers a Q and A room where members can post questions at any time, an archive of webinars, videos, meditations, mindfulness exercises, reflections, 101 gentle reminders, daily challenges and coping tips, all to encourage you.

This site presents you with an experiential immersion in responsible, inspiring, encouraging and supportive content. Over time you will build a resource toolbox that you can access when needed, and this will help you to keep your perspective on healing and guide you on in your recovery journey.

The International Antidepressant Withdrawal Project

www.antidepressantwithdrawal.info
The International Antidepressant Project helps people make a fully informed decision about taking antidepressants; discusses dangers connected with taking them; advises on tapering methods; and supports through withdrawal and recovery.

We offer information and discussion on alternative healing methods; the latest media on medications, Big Pharma, neuroscience, and health; our own educational and informational videos; spiritual and psychic matters; music; humor; and uplifting stories from the news.

International Coalition for Drug Awareness

www.drugawareness.org
"Educating about the dangers of Rx Medications." Includes an Mp3 download: "How to withdraw safely from antidepressant medications

(Details safe and successful withdrawal from antidepressants, benzodiazepines, or any other type of mind-altering medications).

The International Society for Ethical Psychology and Psychiatry, Inc. (ISEPP)

www.psychintegrity.org
A non-profit volunteer organization of mental health professionals, physicians, educators, ex-patients and survivors of the mental health system, and their families. We are not affiliated with any political or religious group.

Our mission is to use the standards of scientific inquiry and critical reasoning to address the ethics of psychology and psychiatry. We strive to educate the public about the nature of "mental illness", the de-humanizing and coercive aspects of many forms of mental health treatment, and the alternative humane ways of helping people who struggle with very difficult life issues.

We believe this is essential since one of the most cherished principles of the mental profession is "informed consent". That means you should be fully and honestly informed about the problems you are experiencing, and the full risks and benefits of any treatment, before making truly voluntary decisions about your care. Our goal is to fully inform you.

The International Institute for Psychiatric Drug Withdrawal

www.iipdw.org
We support the process of reducing and withdrawing from psychiatric drugs through practice, research and training.

AntiDepAware

www.antidepaware.co.uk
Promoting the awareness of the dangers of antidepressants. This website, which I began in 2013, includes links to reports of inquests held in England and Wales since 2003. Most of these were found in the online

archives of local and national newspapers. It must be noted that these lists are far from exhaustive but, even so, contain summaries of more than 7500 reports on self-inflicted deaths, all of which are related to use of antidepressants. There are also many articles, most of which I have written myself, based on what I have discovered during my research. My motivation in embarking on this site has been to offer some understanding to the grieving families who are invariably left a legacy of unanswered questions and "if only's", along with misplaced guilt and the memory of horrific loss. Perhaps this website will help answer some of their questions.

SSRI Stories: Antidepressant Nightmares

www.ssristories.org
SSRI Stories is a collection of over 7,000 stories most of which were published newspapers or scientific journals. In these stories, prescription antidepressant medications are mentioned. Common to all of them is the possibility—sometimes the near certainty—that the drugs caused or were a contributing factor to some negative outcome: suicide, violence, serious physical problems, bad withdrawal reactions, personality change leading to loss of reputation and relationships, etc.

Institute for Safe Medication Practices

www.ismp.org
Educates the healthcare community and consumers about safe medication practices. Includes a mix of resources for free and at a cost.

TaperMD

www.tapermd.com
Leading-Edge Medication Therapy Management and Drug Review Tool TaperMD is a clinically-proven tool—integrating healthcare information for healthcare providers to optimize care decisions and save time. The

patient focused dashboard streamlines visual evidence and review tools to avoid information overload.

Our vision is of a medical system where explicit interventions for reducing the burden of treatment are part of routine preventive care—just like immunization and screening.

TaperMD was originally developed by Data Based Medicine Americas Ltd., in conjunction with the Department of Family Medicine at McMaster University, to help reduce the medication burden in seniors. We have used it in various research studies to validate and improve the system, and now we are offering it for broader clinical use beginning with approved beta testers. For more information on the McMaster Taper project click here.

With TaperMD, patients and their health care professionals have a simple but powerful tool to begin a meaningful conversation by discussing questions such as:

- Do I still need all of my medications or can some of them be tapered or stopped?
- Do my medications reflect my priorities for care?
- Can this effect that I am experiencing be caused by a medication?
- Can my pill regimen be simplified?
- Are there strategies that don't use drugs for my condition?

Open Dialogue

www.dialogicpractice.net

Open Dialogue is an innovative, network-based approach to psychiatric care that was first developed in the 1980s by a multidisciplinary team at Keropudas Hospital in Tornio, Finland. It is a new approach to mental healthcare. In contrast to standard treatments for early psychosis and other crises, Open Dialogue emphasizes listening and understanding and engages the social network from the very beginning—rather than relying solely on medication and hospitalization. It comprises both a way of organizing a treatment system and a form of therapeutic conversation, or Dialogic Practice, within that system.

Everything Matters—Beyond Meds

www.beyondmeds.com
Monica Cassani documents and shares many natural methods of self-care for finding and sustaining health in body, mind and spirit and deals with wider issues in the socio/political and spiritual realms as they pertain to mental health and human rights issues surrounding psychiatry."

Warfighter Advance

www.warfighteradvance.org
Warfighter Advance changes the trajectory of the warfighter's post-deployment life, so that rather than an existence characterized by an endless cycle of mental illness diagnoses, medications, medical appointments and disappointments, the warfighter has a life characterized by pride, productivity, healthy relationships, continued service, and advocacy for the same outcomes for their fellow service members.

A Disorder For Everyone

www.adisorder4everyone.com
Challenging the culture of psychiatric diagnosis. Exploring trauma informed alternatives. We need an altogether different approach to emotional distress than slapping labels onto people that have essentially been made up around a table!

Chaya Grossberg

www.chayagrossberg.com
"Med Free Solutions for a Med FREE Life"

Do you wish there was a magic pill to get off psychiatric medication as quickly as easily as you got on? Do you long for that alive, alert and connected feeling you once had in life?

Do concerns about how to get off psychiatric medication negatively affect your life? Do you feel your doctors inadequately provide the support you really need? You're in the right place. I have helped many successfully get off psychiatric medication, and reclaim their energy, health, and life. And I can help YOU. I'm not a magic pill. But I can help you see and clarify your purpose. I can help provide healthy and holistic alternatives to help you get off psychiatric medication so you can have your life back. Together we can map out the road back to freedom. I offer my story, how I was able to get off psychiatric medication, and tried and true methods.

Emotional CPR

www.emotional-cpr.org

Emotional CPR (eCPR) is an educational program designed to teach people to assist others through an emotional crisis by three simple steps: C = Connecting P = emPowering, and R = Revitalizing.

The Connecting process of eCPR involves deepening listening skills, practicing presence, and creating a sense of safety for the person experiencing a crisis. The emPowering process helps people better understand how to feel empowered themselves as well as to assist others to feel more hopeful and engaged in life. In the Revitalizating process, people re-engage in relationships with their loved ones or their support system, and they resume or begin routines that support health and wellness which reinforces the person's sense of mastery and accomplishment, further energizing the healing process.

eCPR is based on the principles found to be shared by a number of support approaches: trauma-informed care, counseling after disasters, peer support to avoid continuing emotional despair, emotional intelligence, suicide prevention, and cultural attunement. It was developed with input from a diverse cadre of recognized leaders from across the U.S., who themselves have learned how to recover and grow from emotional crises. They have wisdom by the grace of first-hand experience."

Integrative Mental Health for You

www.imhu.org

- Learn about effective alternatives to psychiatric medications in online presentations Understand phenomena of spiritual awakening
- Find out how to manage spiritual crisis We specialize in
- Cultivating Spiritual Emergence
- An Integrative Approach to Mental Health
- Unique Courses and Continuing Ed credits available for health care providers

The OLLIE Foundation

www.theolliefoundation.org

OLLIE is a charity dedicated to delivering suicide awareness, intervention and prevention training by empowering professionals and young adults in their own communities to lead suicide prevention activities. It is widely accepted in society that with appropriate support and education, suicide can be prevented.

We do this by:

- Providing confidential help and advice to young people and anyone worried about a young person
- Helping others to prevent young suicide by delivering a number of training programs
- Campaigning and influencing national policy

Human Givens

www.hgi.org.uk
Thousands of people around the world recognize that the organizing ideas summed up in the phrase 'human givens' have enormous, beneficial implications for education, mental health, social order and the world of business, politics and diplomacy. The human givens approach enables us to think more clearly about a wide range of social issues to do with the running of society and the future and physical survival of our species, including how we bring up children to live in a rapidly changing environment.

Compassionate Mental Health

www.compassionatementalhealth.co.uk
Compassionate Mental Health is working with a network of people across the UK and internationally to transform mental health services, and radically change the conversation around mental illness. OUR VISION is of a world where more people recover after a serious mental health crisis, and people have access to a range of compassionate services to help develop positive mental health and wellbeing.

The Icarus Project

www.ibpf.org
The Icarus Project envisions a new culture and language that resonates with our actual experiences of 'mental illness' rather than trying to fit our lives into a conventional framework. We are a network of people living with and/or affected by experiences that are commonly diagnosed and labeled as psychiatric conditions. We believe these experiences are mad gifts needing cultivation and care, rather than diseases or disorders. By joining together as individuals and as a community, the intertwined threads of madness, creativity, and collaboration can inspire hope and transformation in an oppressive and damaged world.

Epidemic Answers

www.epidemicanswers.org
Unacceptable numbers of children are ill, impaired, delayed and struggling while caregivers feel overwhelmed, misinformed, and disempowered in a culture and system that neither fully values their inherent wisdom and authority nor respects the interdependence of human and planetary health.

Our vision is a world where parents and professionals are empowered with the knowledge, resources and support essential to raising healthy and vibrant children in today's world.

Our mission is to generate and share essential knowledge, inspire innovation, and build community in order to prevent and reverse children's chronic health and developmental conditions so they may thrive in today's world.

UK Post SSRI Sexual Dysfunction Organization

www.pssd-uk.org
We are an association for people in the UK experiencing an iatrogenic (meaning caused by a medication or medical treatment) disorder known commonly as Post-SSRI Sexual Dysfunction or Post SSRI/SNRI Sexual Dysfunction. This disorder arises during or after the use of SSRI (selective serotonin re-uptake inhibitor) and SNRI (Serotonin-norepinephrine re-uptake inhibitor) antidepressants. Though characterized by a reduction or removal of sexual functioning, common symptoms also include emotional blunting, cognitive dysfunction, genital numbness and other symptoms. The causes of PSSD are poorly understood and there are no known reliable treatments. The disorder can arise from brief exposure to SSRIs or SNRIs and can persist for months, years or indefinitely. Though recognized by the European Medicines Agency, PSSD is not yet officially acknowledged by the Department of Health, the NHS or NICE guidelines. The association and website exist to bring together people in the UK suffering from this condition and advocate

for recognition, research and greater transparency within psychiatry concerning the risks of antidepressants.

Antidepressant Risks: Helping People Understand the Risks of Taking Antidepressants

www.antidepressantrisks.org

The aims of this site are:

- To share stories of people who have been harmed by antidepressants and other depression medications. See Stolen Lives.
- To make people aware of the side effects of antidepressants and the difficulty of withdrawal.
- To explain that adverse reactions to antidepressants can cause suicide, violence and homicide.
- To draw attention to the potentially life threatening conditions of serotonin syndrome and akathisia.

We are a team of people with experience of these drugs and with access to experts. We have come together to share our knowledge and experience to help people understand the risks of taking antidepressants.

Canada Post SSRI Sexual Dysfunction Organization

www.pssdcanada.cd

We are a group of Canadians experiencing an iatrogenic (meaning caused by a medication or medical treatment) disorder known commonly as Post-SSRI Sexual Dysfunction or Post SSRI/SNRI Sexual Dysfunction. This disorder arises during or after the use of SSRI (selective serotonin re-uptake inhibitor) and SNRI (Serotonin-norepinephrine re-uptake inhibitor) antidepressants. Though characterized by a reduction or removal of sexual functioning, common symptoms also include emotional blunting, cognitive dysfunction, genital numbness and sleep disruption. The causes of PSSD are poorly understood and there are no known reliable treatments. The disorder can arise from brief exposure to

SSRIs or SNRIs and can persist for months, years or indefinitely. This page exists to bring together people in Canada suffering from this condition and advocate for recognition, research and greater transparency within psychiatry concerning the risks of antidepressants.

Critical Psychiatry Network

www.criticalpsychiatry.co.uk
Critical psychiatry is a broad critique of mainstream psychiatry that has emerged in recent years which challenges some of psychiatry's most deeply held assumptions. It mounts a scientific challenge to claims about the nature and causes of mental disorder and the effects of psychiatric interventions, and draws on philosophy, history, anthropology, social science and mental health service users' experiences. There is no definitive 'critical psychiatry position.' It is a collection of critical perspectives intended to produce a more reflective, skeptical and patient-centered approach to the theory and practice of psychiatry.

www.Woodymatters.com

www.kimwitczak.com
Kim Witczak is a leading global drug safety advocate and speaker with over 25 years professional experience in advertising and marketing communications. She became involved in pharmaceutical drug safety issues after the sudden death of her husband due to undisclosed drug side effect of an antidepressant. Kim co-founded Woodymatters, a non-profit dedicated to advocating for a stronger FDA and drug safety system. She co-created and organized the international, multi-disciplinary conference Selling Sickness: People Before Profits conference in Washington, D.C.

ADDITIONAL READING

A Mind of Your Own: The Truth About Depression and How Women Can Heal Their Bodies to Reclaim Their Lives by Kelly Brogan, MD with Kristin Loberg

A Straight-Talking Introduction to Psychiatric Diagnosis by Lucy Johnstone

A Straight-Talking Introduction to Psychiatric Drugs (Second Edition): The Truth About How They Work And How To Come Off Them by Joanna Moncrieff

A Straight-Talking Introduction to Caring for Someone with Mental Health Problems by Jen Kilyon and Theresa Smith

A Straight-Talking Introduction to Children's Mental Health Problems by Sami Timimi

A Straight-Talking Introduction to the Causes of Mental Health Problems by John Read and Pete Sanders

ADHD Nation: Children, Doctors, Big Pharma, and the Making of an American Epidemic by Alan Schwarz

Alternatives Beyond Psychiatry by Peter Stastny and Peter Lehmann

Anatomy of an Epidemic: Magic Bullets, Psychiatric Drugs, and the Astonishing Rise of Mental Illness in America by Robert Whitaker

Being Old Is Different: Person-Centred Care For Old People by Marlis Pörtner

Bottle of Lies: The Inside Story of the Generic Drug Boom by Katherine Eban

Can Medicine Be Cured?: The Corruption of a Profession by Seamus O'Mahony

Coming Off Psychiatric Drugs by Peter Lehmann

Cracked: Why Psychiatry is Doing More Harm Than Good by James Davies

Crazy Like Us: The Globalization of the American Psyche by Ethan Watters

Deadly Medicines and Organized Crime by Peter Gøtzsche

Depression Delusion by Dr. Terry Lynch

Drop The Disorder! Challenging The Culture Of Psychiatric Diagnosis by Jo Watson

Emperor's New Drugs: Exploding the Antidepressant Myth by Irving Kirsch

Generic: The Unbranding of Modern Medicine by Jeremy A. Greene

Guidance for Psychological Therapists: Enabling Conversations with Clients Taking or Withdrawing From Prescribed Psychiatric Drugs (www.prescribeddrug.info)

Harm Reduction Guide to Coming off Psychiatric Drugs (Second Edition) by Will Hall Icarus Project and Freedom Centre

Insane Medicine by Sami Timimi

Inside Out, Outside In: Transforming Mental Health Practices by Lydia Sapouna, Harry Gijbels and Gary Sidley

It's Not Always Depression: Working the Change Triangle to Listen to the Body, Discover Core Emotions, and Connect to Your Authentic Self by Hilary Jacobs Hendel and Diana Fosha

JCPCP The Journal of Critical Psycholgy, Counselling and Psychotherapy, Volume 20, #4 Winter 2020, Special Edition: Withdrawal from Prescribed Drugs

Lost Connections: Why You're Depressed and How to Find Hope by Johann Hari

Mad in America: Bad Science, Bad Medicine, and the Enduring Mistreatment of the Mentally Ill by Robert Whitaker

Mad Medicine: Myths, Maxims and Mayhem in the National Health Service by Dr Andrew Bamji

Mad Science: Psychiatric Coercion, Diagnosis, and Drugs By Stuart A. Kirk, Tomi Gomory, and David Cohen

Madness Explained Psychosis and Human Nature by Richard P. Bentall

Malcharist by Paul John Scott

Mental Health, Inc.: How Corruption, Lax Oversight and Failed Reforms Endanger Our Most Vulnerable Citizens by Art Levine

Own Your Self: The Surprising Path beyond Depression, Anxiety, and Fatigue to Reclaiming Your Authenticity, Vitality, and Freedom by Kelly Brogan, MD

Psychiatric Drug Withdrawal: A Guide for Prescribers, Therapists, Patients and their Families by Peter R. Breggin

Psychiatric Drugs Key Issues and Service Users Perspectives by Jim Read

Psychiatry and Mental Health: A Guide for Counsellors and Psychotherapists by Rachel Freeth

Psychiatry and The Business of Madness by Bonnie Burstow

Psychiatry Under The Influence: Institutional Corruption, Social Injury, and Prescriptions for Reform by Robert Whitaker and Lisa Cosgrove

Saving Normal: An Insider's Revolt Against Out-of-Control Psychiatric Diagnosis, DSM-5, Big Pharma, and the Medicalization of Ordinary Life by Allen Frances, MD

Sedated: How Modern Capitalism Created Our Mental Health Crisis by James Davies

The Antidepressant Solution: A Step by Step Guide to Safely Overcoming Antidepressant Withdrawal, Dependence, and Addiction by Joseph Glenmullen, MD

The Body Keeps the Score Brain, Mind, and Body in the Healing of Trauma by Bessel Van Der Kolk, MD

The Patient Revolution: How We Can Heal the Healthcare System by David Gilbert

Mental Health, Inc.: How Corruption, Lax Oversight and Failed Reforms Endanger Our Most Vulnerable Citizens by Art Levine

Own Your Self: The Surprising Path beyond Depression, Anxiety, and Fatigue to Reclaiming Your Authenticity, Vitality, and Freedom by Kelly Brogan, MD

Psychiatric Drug Withdrawal: A Guide for Prescribers, Therapists, Patients and their Families by Peter R. Breggin

Psychiatry and Mental Health: A Guide for Counsellors and Psychotherapists by Rachel Freeth

Psychiatry Under The Influence: Institutional Corruption, Social Injury, and Prescriptions for Reform by Robert Whitaker and Lisa Cosgrove

Saving Normal: An Insider's Revolt Against Out-of-Control Psychiatric Diagnosis, DSM-5, Big Pharma, and the Medicalization of Ordinary Life by Allen Frances, MD

Sedated: How Modern Capitalism Created Our Mental Health Crisis by James Davies

The Body Keeps the Score Brain, Mind, and Body in the Healing of Trauma by Bessel Van Der Kolk, MD

The Pill That Steals Lives: One Woman's Terrifying Journey to Discover the Truth about Antidepressants by Katinka Blackford Newman

The Truth about the Drug Companies: How They Deceive Us and What to Do About It by Marsha Angell, MD

The Zyprexa Papers by Jim Gottstein

They Say You're Crazy: How The World's Most Powerful Psychiatrists Decide Who's Normal by Paula Caplan

Toxic Psychiatry: Why Therapy, Empathy and Love Must Replace the Drugs, Electroshock, and Biochemical Theories of the "New Psychiatry" by Peter Breggin

When the Body Says No: The Cost of Hidden Stress by Gabor Maté, MD

Your Drug May Be Your Problem: How and Why to Stop Taking Psychiatric Medications by Peter Breggin and David Cohen

KEY ARTICLES, INFORMATION AND RESEARCH

Informed Consent and Prescribing

www.fda.gov/regulatory-information/search-fda-guidance-documents/informed-consent

apa.org/monitor/2012/06/prescribing

theinnercompass.org/blog

www.gmc-uk.org/ethical-guidance/ethical-guidance-for-doctors/decision-making-and-consent

www.counterpunch.org/2014/05/14/psychiatrys-manufacture-of-consent

bigthink.com/surprising-science/antidepressant-effects

popularresistance.org/psychiatrys-manufacture-of-consent-the-antidepressant-explosion

doi.org/10.1136/bmj.n895

bjgplife.com/2021/04/20/the-four-research-papers-i-wish-my-doctor-had-read-before-prescribing-an-antidepressant/?fbclid=IwAR3x-h79cEDzg2viPUYXVmvzHcUhkMkcjhX8qmrDlHyjaTadbsAlPYv_BFI

Withdrawal/Tapering

Lewis, S. (2021). The four research papers I wish my doctor had read before prescribing an antidepressant. *British Journal of Medical Practice.* DOI: doi.org/10.3399/bjgp21X716321

www.madinamerica.com/2021/07/223158

www.cochranelibrary.com/cdsr/doi/10.1002/14651858.CD013495.pub2/full

withdrawal.theinnercompass.org/taper/determine-how-taper-friendly-your-drug

withdrawal.theinnercompass.org/learn/psychiatric-drug-taper-rates-review-and-discussion

withdrawal.theinnercompass.org/page/withdrawal-symptoms-z rxisk.org/guide-stopping-antidepressants

survivingantidepressants.org/forum/14-tapering

survivingantidepressants.org/topic/9167-how-to-calculate-dosages-and-dilutions-spreadsheets-and-calculators

nytimes.com/2019/03/05/health/depression-withdrawal-drugs.html

psychologytoday.com/us/blog/sideeffects/201810/antidepressant-withdrawal-said-affect-millions

rcpsych.ac.uk/mental-health/treatments-and-wellbeing/stopping-antidepressants

pharmaceutical-journal.com/news-and-analysis/news/national-guidance-for-antidepressant-withdrawal-too-fast-for-some-patients-says-rcpsych/20206614.article?firstPass=false

thelancet.com/article/S2215-0366(19)30032-X/fulltext

rcpsych.ac.uk/mental-health/treatments-and-wellbeing/stopping-antidepressants

apa.org/monitor/2020/04/stop-antidepressants

pubmed.ncbi.nlm.nih.gov/32435449

www.antidepressantsfacts.com/effexor-withdrawal6.htm

nytimes.com/2011/07/10/opinion/sunday/10antidepressants.html?pagewanted=all

psychologytoday.com/us/blog/sideeffects/201107/antidepressant-withdrawal-syndrome

pubmed.ncbi.nlm.nih.gov/30292574

cambridge.org/core/journals/epidemiology-and-psychiatric-sciences/article/antidepressant-withdrawal-the-tide-is-finally-turning/8394C10FE317CA5A39B62B86793FC3ED

psychologytoday.com/us/blog/sideeffects/201908/antidepressant-withdrawal-and-scientific-consensus

madinamerica.com/2020/01/researchers-antidepressant-withdrawal-not-discontinuation-syndrome

psychiatrictimes.com/view/international-antidepressant-withdrawal-crisis-time-act

bma.org.uk/what-we-do/population-health/prescription-and-illicit-drugs/prescribed-drugs-associated-with-dependence-and-withdrawal

thelancet.com/journals/lanpsy/article/PIIS2215-0366(19)30032-X/fulltext

bpspubs.onlinelibrary.wiley.com/doi/full/10.1111/bcp.14475

bpspubs.onlinelibrary.wiley.com/doi/10.1111

southampton.ac.uk/medicine/academic_units/projects/reduce.page#project_overview%0A

preprints.jmir.org/preprint/25537/submitted

medicine.unimelb.edu.au/research-groups/general-practice-research/mental-health-program/wiserad-a-randomised-trial-of-a-structured-online-intervention-to-promote-and-support-antidepressant-de-prescribing-in-primary-care
umcg.nl/EN/corporate/News/Paginas/first-patient-discontinuation-antidepressants.aspx

madinamerica.com/2013/08/ssri-discontinuation-is-even-more-problematic-than-acknowledged rxisk.org/protracted-antidepressant-withdrawal

psychiatryonline.org/pb/assets/raw/sitewide/practice_guidelines/guidelines/mdd.pdf

michaelwest.com.au/websites-research-online-advice-on-medications-skewed-by-big-pharma-funding

content.iospress.com/articles/international-journal-of-risk-and-safety-in-medicine/jrs191023

americanaddictioncenters.org/withdrawal-timelines-treatments/anti-depressants

bjgp.org/content/early/2021/04/19/BJGP.2020.0913?fbclid=IwAR0YkYvgtAY_WWj63LUOkLvp3dijcyGQJvlFALz7NEayFzTMgrzhwwWLeYQ#ref-25

journals.sagepub.com/doi/10.1177/2045125320980573

journals.sagepub.com/doi/full/10.1177/2045125321991274

DOI: doi.org/10.1136/bmj.n1065; "Antidepressants: Evidence on safe discontinuation is lacking, concludes Cochrane review". BMJ 2021; 373.

www.theguardian.com/commentisfree/2021/may/17/antidepressant-use-up-covid-side-effects-medication

www.newyorker.com/magazine/2019/04/08/the-challenge-of-going-off-psychiatric-drugs

connect.springerpub.com/content/sgrehpp/early/2021/01/12/ehpp-d-20-00006

pharmaceutical-journal.com/article/news/nice-amends-depression-guideline-highlighting-severe-and-long-lasting-withdrawal-symptoms

www.pulsetoday.co.uk/news/clinical-areas/prescribing/nice-antidepressant-withdrawal-guidance-misleading-and-without-evidence

Patient Experiences

parliament.scot/GettingInvolved/Petitions/PE01651

petitions.senedd.wales/petitions/1235

survivingantidepressants.org/forum/28-success-stories-recovery-from-withdrawal

blogs.bmj.com/bmj/2013/12/04/kelly-brendel-experiences-of-antidepressants-everyone-has-a-story-to-tell/

theguardian.com/society/2013/nov/21/your-experiences-antidepressants-responses

byrdie.com/antidepressant-stories

www.hgi.org.uk/resources/delve-our-extensive-library/case-histories/case-study-antidepressant-experience

nami.org/Personal-Stories/How-Antidepressants-Saved-My-Life

ncbi.nlm.nih.gov/books/NBK361002/

Coming off Psych Drugs: A meeting of the Minds

wildtruth.net/films-english/psychdrugs/Medicating Normal

medicatingnormal.com

www.madinamerica.com/2020/10/insane-medicine-chapter-one

Report Your Withdrawal Experience

USA
accessdata.fda.gov/scripts/medwatch/index.cfm?action=reporting.home

Canada
hpr-rps.hres.ca/sideeffects-reporting-form.php?form=voluntary

Guidelines for Switching From One Antidepressant to Another

withdrawal.theinnercompass.org/taper/reflections-switch-or-not-switch

cks.nice.org.uk/topics/depression/prescribing-information/switching-antidepressants

nps.org.au/assets/Products/Guidelines-switching-antidepressants_A3.pdf

www.members.wokinghamccg.nhs.uk/images/docman-files/southreading/SRCCGTIPS/SRTIPS%2017May2017/GP%20TIPS%2017May2017/Swapping%20and%20stopping%20antidepressants.pdf

Tapering Strips

taperingstrip.com

thelancet.com/journals/lanpsy/article/PIIS2215-0366(19)30032-X/fulltext

.pharmaceutical-journal.com/news-and-analysis/opinion/insight/antidepressant-withdrawal-can-be-a-horrible-experience-are-tapering-strips-a-potential-solution/20207867.fullarticle?firstPass=false

Adverse Effects

madinamerica.com/2016/11/whats-harm-taking-antidepressant

rxisk.org/experiencing-a-drug-side-effect

washingtonpost.com/national/health-science/doctors-often-dont-tell-you-about-drug-side effects-and-thats-a-problem/2017/07/28/830fbaf6-715c-11e7-8839-ec48ec4cae25_story.html

hormonesmatter.com/brain-long-term-lexapro-chemically-induced-tbi

breggin.com/studies/Breggin2007.pdf

psycom.net/serotonin-syndrome

rxisk.org/post-ssri-sexual-dysfunction-pssd

health.harvard.edu/womens-health/when-an-ssri-medication-impacts-your-sex-life

rxisk.org/wp-content/uploads/2015/02/2014-Brookwell-SSRIs-and-Alcohol-JRS616.pdf

pubmed.ncbi.nlm.nih.gov/23796469

rxisk.org/driven-to-drink-antidepressants-and-cravings-for-alcohol

madinamerica.com/wp-content/uploads/2017/01/Age-of-Prozac.pdf

rxisk.org/the-dark-is-for-mushrooms-not-for-women

health.usnews.com/health-news/patient-advice/articles/2016-01-13/antidepressants-during-pregnancy-stay-on-them-or-stop

cdc.gov/pregnancy/meds/treatingfortwo/features/ssrisandbirthdefects.html

healthline.com/health-news/do-antidepressants-help-in-long-run#Conclusions-are-tough-to-draw

cepuk.org/unrecognised-facts/long-term-outcomes/

pdfs.semanticscholar.org/c280/181ab5a63ad93dfdc090eace0d3e0865b6c4.pdf

dovepress.com/long-term-antidepressant-use-patient-perspectives-of-benefits-and-adve-peer-reviewed-article-PPA

news.sky.com/story/long-term-use-of-antidepressants-could-cause-permanent-damage-doctors-warn-11688430

journals.sagepub.com/doi/full/10.1177/2045125320921694

Breggin P R, 2011,Psychiatric drug induced Chronic Brain Impairment (CBI): Implications for long term treatment with psychiatric medication, International Journal of Risk & Safety in Medicine, 23: 193-200)

ncbi.nlm.nih.gov/pmc/articles/PMC5347943/?fbclid=IwAR1B6cNzk vCPBR wQyI8VxbDSxHIq45R82jqeTLgNjhRDrrr3-qPR-VUXTG8

bmj.com/content/361/bmj.k1315

uk.finance.yahoo.com/news/antidepressants-taken-millions-significantly-increase-dementia-risk-

pubmed.ncbi.nlm.nih.gov/24502860

care.diabetesjournals.org/content/early/2020/02/12/dc19-1175

madnessradio.net/files/tardivedysphoriadarticle.pdf psychologytoday.com/us/blog/mad-in-america/201106/now-antidepressant-induced-chronic-depression-has-name-tardive-dysphoria midcitiespsychiatry.com/treatment-resistant-depression

pubmed.ncbi.nlm.nih.gov/22654508

en.wikipedia.org/wiki/Antidepressant_treatment_tachyphylaxis

healthyplace.com/depression/antidepressants/do-antidepressants-lose-their-effect

Akathisia

akathisiaalliance.org

missd.co

davidhealy.org/left-hanging-suicide-in-bridgend

rxisk.org/illnesses-worse-than-side effects

rxisk.org/akathisia

akathisiainfo.wordpress.com/2012/03/10/akathisia-info

Dependence

withdrawal.theinnercompass.org/learn/primer-psychiatric-drug-dependence-tolerance-and-withdrawal

drugabuse.gov/publications/media-guide/science-drug-use-addiction-basics

nytimes.com/2018/04/07/health/antidepressants-withdrawal-prozac-cymbalta.html

bma.org.uk/what-we-do/population-health/prescription-and-illicit-drugs/prescribed-drugs-associated-with-dependence-and-withdrawal

health.harvard.edu/blog/millions-skip-medications-due-to-their-high-cost-201501307673

thenation.com/article/society/mental-health-insurance-coronavirus

ctvnews.ca/health/canadians-warn-of-self-harm-risk-amid-severe-shortage-of-antidepressant-drug-1.5200797

Drug Interactions

drugs.com/drug_interactions.html

www.rxisk.org/tools/guides

rxisk.org/tools/drug-interaction-checker

www.smartcarebhcs.org/important-drug-interactions-with-the-ssris

Antidepressants and Suicide

www.antidepaware.co.uk

fda.gov/media/72995/download

accessdata.fda.gov/drugsatfda_docs/label/2012/020151s059,020699s100mg.pdf ncbi.nlm.nih.gov/pmc/articles/PMC2771172

sciencedaily.com/releases/2004/12/041203100252.htm karger.com/Article/Pdf/501215

breggin.com/violence-and-suicide-caused-by-antidepressants-report-to-the-fda

ncbi.nlm.nih.gov/pmc/articles/PMC5061092

dx.doi.org/10.15585/mmwr.mm6722a1

weforum.org/agenda/2019/05/the-global-suicide-rate-is-growing-what-can-we-do

ncbi.nlm.nih.gov/pubmed/19610491

www.ssristories.org

nytimes.com/2020/05/19/health/pandemic-coronavirus-suicide-health.html fda.gov/media/72995/download accessdata.fda.gov/drugsatfda_docs/label/2012/020151s059,020699s100mg.pdf

Overprescribing

www.heraldscotland.com/news/19256645.no-good-evidence-long-term-use-antidepressants

nytimes.com/2020/09/07/well/live/prescription-medication-drug-side effects-cascade.html

washingtonpost.com/national/health-science/doctors-often-dont-tell-you-about-drug-side effects-and-thats-a-problem/2017/07/28/830fbaf6-715c-11e7-8839-ec48ec4cae25_story.html

www.bbc.co.uk/news/uk-wales-56087135

pimsplus.org/about

Medically Unexplained Symptoms

bjgplife.com/2021/05/19/a-50-year-timeline-including-the-1990s-defeat-depression-campaign

en.wikipedia.org/wiki/Medically_unexplained_physical_symptoms

bjgplife.com/2020/12/03/the-patient-voice-antidepressant-withdrawal-mus-and-fnd

hulpgids.nl/assets/files/pdf/DESS.pdf

ncbi.nlm.nih.gov/pmc/articles/PMC4820447

ncbi.nlm.nih.gov/pmc/articles/PMC5864293

apa.org/monitor/2013/07-08/symptoms

bmj.com/content/346/bmj.f1580

bmj.com/content/346/bmj.f1580/rapid-responses

providers.bcidaho.com/resources/pdfs/medical-management/behavioral-health/PHQ-15.pdf

hgi.org.uk/sites/default/files/hgi/Marions%20infographic_for%20print%20A4%20x%202%20pages.pdf

Generics

statista.com/statistics/205042/proportion-of-brand-to-generic-prescriptions-dispensed

Rosenthal, Jessica & Kong, Brian & Jacobs, Leslie & Katzman, Martin. (2008) The Journal of family practice. 57. 109-14.

www.psychiatrictimes.com/view/antidepressants-brand-name-or-generic

The Role of Relatives and Friends in Antidepressant Treatment

d3hgrlq6yacptf.cloudfront.net/5f44fd4229433/content/pages/documents/1490101 072.pdf

Drug Interactions

drugs.com/drug_interactions.html

rxisk.org/tools/guides

rxisk.org/tools/drug-interaction-checker/

www.smartcarebhcs.org/important-drug-interactions-with-the-ssris

Antidepressants and Young People

www.thestar.com/news/investigations/2021/04/26/more-kids-on-antidepressants-in-canada-than-ever-before-prescribing-doctors-say-they-have-little-choice-as-youth-cant-wait-nine-months-for-therapy.html

newstatesman.com/spotlight/healthcare/2020/05/why-mental-health-human-right

Selective serotonin reuptake inhibitors in childhood depression. Whittington, C. The Lancet 363 (2004):1341-5.

www.bbc.co.uk/news/uk-scotland-42917452

fda.gov/drugs/postmarket-drug-safety-information-patients-and-providers/suicidality-children-and-adolescents-being-treated-antidepressant-medications

fda.gov/consumers/consumer-updates/fda-dont-leave-childhood-depression-untreated

fda.gov/drugs/postmarket-drug-safety-information-patients-and-providers/suicidality-children-and-adolescents-being-treated-antidepressant-medications

verywellmind.com/should-children-take-antidepressants-2330670 info.1in5minds.org/blog/7-free-screening-tools-for-childrens-mental-health-concerns#

madinamerica.com/antidepressants-pediatric-use

ews.curtin.edu.au/media-releases/research-reveals-alarming-link-between-rising-antidepressant-use-and-suicide-rates-among-young-australians

wix.app/blog/post/5f98d1f2b616490017b79f82?metaSiteId=e46126be-5e83-4973-a0fe-598613447990&d=psychwatchaustralia.com/post/melbourne-s-covid-spike-in-antidepressant-use-may-trigger-suicides-by-children-and-ado lescents?postId%3D5f98d1f2b616490017b79f82

A. Martin. "Age effects on antidepressant-induced manic conversion," Arch of Pediatrics & Adolescent Medicine(2002) 158: 773-80

www.theguardian.com/society/2018/nov/25/young-people-are-being-prescribed-dangerous-antidepressants

Antidepressants and the Elderly

bpac.org.nz/BPJ/2010/April/stopguide.aspx

Bartels, Stephen et al. Evidence-Based Practices in Geriatric Mental Health in Psychiatric Services, November 2002. www.ps.psychiatryonline.org/cgi/content/full/53/11/1419

Arthur, A., Savva, G. M., Barnes, L. E., Borjian-Boroojeny, A., Dening, T., Jagger, C., & The Cognitive Function and Ageing Studies Collaboration. (2019). Changing prevalence and treatment of depression among older people over two decades. The British Journal of Psychiatry. DOI: 10.1192/bjp.2019.193

bmj.com/content/343/bmj.d4551 Coupland, Carol et al. "Antidepressant use and risk of adverse outcomes in older people: population based cohort study" in BMJ, August 2, 2011.

www.bmj.com/content/343/bmj.d4551

Weigand AJ, Bondi MW, Thomas KR, Campbell NL, Galasko DR, Salmon DP, & Delano-Wood L. (2020). Association of anticholinergic medication and AD biomarkers with incidence of MCI among cognitively normal older adults. Neurology. Published online September 2, 2020. DOI: 10.1212/WNL.0000000000010643

DLinx (January 2019). mdlinx.com/internal-medicine/article/3272. psychologytoday.com/us/blog/envy/201902/loneliness-new-epidemic-in-the-usa

nia.nih.gov/health/depression-and-older-adults

Antidepressants and Veterans

warfighteradvance.org

ncbi.nlm.nih.gov/pmc/articles/PMC5047000/ ptsd.va.gov/professional/assessment/screens/pc-ptsd.asp

madinamerica.com/2019/11/screening-drug-treatment-increase-veteran-suicides

washingtonpost.com/opinions/2020/09/17/im-veteran-who-was-suicidal-its-good-thing-i-didnt-have-access-gun

huffingtonpost.co.uk/entry/veterans-ptsd-marijuana_n_7506760?ri18n=true

madinamerica.com/veterans-2

Social Media Support Groups

Facebook has numerous antidepressant support groups.

Counseling/Psychotherapy

Guy A, Davies J, Rizq R. Guidance for psychological therapists: enabling conversations with clients taking or withdrawing from prescribed psychiatric drugs London APPG for Prescribed Drug Dependence 2019

prescribeddrug.info

ACKNOWLEDGMENTS

I WROTE THIS BOOK in the hope it will help people make informed decisions about antidepressants and change how they think about and treat their "mental health".

There are many people around the world who work tirelessly to raise awareness of the harm caused by antidepressants. There are so many advocates and campaigners I am constantly learning from and whose tenacity and strength never ceases to amaze me. Many of you have dedicated your lives to preventing harm and raising awareness of this issue whilst often living with the devastating effects these drugs have had. This book reflects so much of your amazing work. I thank you all.

In particular, many thanks to my good and trusted friend and associate Marion Brown. I will be forever grateful for your constant support. Your Petition, challenging the Scottish Government to recognize and address the issue of prescribed drug harm and dependence is an amazing example of the power of the patient voice. Thank you also to Dr. Peter Gordon and Dr. Sian Gordon, for your valuable friendship and advice.

My gratitude to Dainius Pūras for his words of support and to Will Hall, James Moore, Jill Nickens, Marion Brown and Sian Gordon for taking the time to read *Antidepressed* and comment. Thanks to Daniel Brummitt for his contribution to the book cover.

This book is for those of you who are suffering and those who have suffered. I would like to thank the many individuals who submitted to the Scottish Petition and told of their often life changing experiences in the hope it would help others. I hope your voices will now be heard and listened to around the world. This book would not be the same without you.

I dedicate *Antidepressed* to the memory of Antony Schofield and the unknown and growing number or people whose lives have been cut short or harmed by antidepressants "taken as prescribed".

Finally, but not least, thanks to my husband David for your constant encouragement, belief in me, and unfaltering support. I couldn't have done it without you.

REFERENCES

INTRODUCTION

1. https://en.wikipedia.org/wiki/Wicked_problem
2 https://www.madinamerica.com/2020/07/latest-un-report-calls-paradigm-shift-mental-health-care-globally/
3. https://undocs.org/A/HRC/44/48
4. United Nations. (2017, June 6). World needs "revolution" in mental health care—UN rights expert. Retrieved May 25, 2020, from OHCHR: http://www.ohchr.org/EN/NewsEvents/Pages/DisplayNews.aspx?NewsID=21689&LangID=E

   https://www.ohchr.org/en/NewsEvents/Pages/DisplayNews.aspx?NewsID=21689&LangID=E
5. https://www.cdc.gov/mentalhealth/learn/index.htm
6. https://www.cdc.gov/nchs/products/databriefs/db377.htm
7. https://www.benefitspro.com/2020/04/23/covid-19-pandemic-sparking-increase-in-antidepressant-use/?slreturn=20201007080253
8. https://mhanational.org/issues/mental-health-america-printed-reports
9. https://www.newsweek.com/americans-are-taking-34-percent-more-anxiety-meds-since-coronavirus-pandemic-started-study-says-1498189
10. https://psychiatryonline.org/pb/assets/raw/sitewide/practice_guidelines/guidelines/mdd.pdf
11. https://adaa.org/finding-help/treatment/low-cost-treatment
12. https://www.aamc.org/news-insights/addressing-escalating-psychiatrist-shortage
13. https://www.madinamerica.com/2017/06/episode-15-robert-whitaker/
14. https://www.ncbi.nlm.nih.gov/pmc/articles/PMC1313341/pdf/10326259.pdf
15. https://www.collaborativemedconsulting.com/single-post/2020/04/10/Mental-illness-is-not-a-disease-and-therefore-cannot-be-an-epidemic-but-unless-we-challenge-the-current-mental-health-narrative-%E2%80%98Memories-of-times-past-will-speak-to-the-present-and-project-on-to-the-unknown-future

PART 1

16. https://www.thedsm5.com/the-dsm-5/
17. https://www.christopherlane.org/critics-blast-the-book-on-mental-illness/
18. http://cepuk.org/unrecognised-facts/diagnostic-system-lacks-validity/
19. http://cepuk.org/unrecognised-facts/regulator-funded-by-industry/
20. https://www.narconon.org/blog/fda-pharma-companies-and-addiction.html
21. https://publications.parliament.uk/pa/cm200405/cmselect/cmhealth/42/4202.htm
22. http://cepuk.org/unrecognised-facts/regulator-funded-by-industry/
23. https://publications.parliament.uk/pa/cm200405/cmselect/cmhealth/42/4210.htm
24. https://www.spravato.com/
25. https://www.medscape.com/viewarticle/921248
26. https://www.thelancet.com/journals/lanpsy/article/PIIS2215-0366(19)30394-3/fulltext
27. https://ajp.psychiatryonline.org/doi/pdfplus/10.1176/ajp.154.6.59
28. https://www.biopsychiatry.com/fluoxetine/prozac-review.html
29. https://marketing-case-studies.blogspot.com/2008/10/prozac-print-campaign.html
30. http://content.time.com/time/magazine/article/0,9171,407338,00.html
31. http://cepuk.org/unrecognised-facts/myth-of-the-chemical-imbalance
32. https://www.counterpunch.org/2014/05/14/psychiatrys-manufacture-of-consent/
33. https://www.psychiatry.org/patients-families/depression/what-is-depression
34. https://www.sciencedaily.com/terms/psychoactive_drug.htm
35. http://www.drugawareness.org/i-am-alarmed-at-the-monster-ssrisnri-antidepressants-i-created-dr-candace-pert/www.bloomberg.com/news/articles/2001-07-22/eli-lilly-life-after-prozac
36. S. Hyman, "Initiation and adaptation: A paradigm for understanding psychotropic drug action," Am J Psychiatry 153 (1996):151-61.
37. http://cepuk.org/unrecognised-facts/altered-mental-states/
38. https://www.bmj.com/content/371/bmj.m3745/rr
39. Boccio M, et al. 'Serotonin, Amygdala & Fear' 2016 https://www.ncbi.nlm.nih.gov/pmc/articles/PMC4820447/

40. Breggin P. 'Neurotoxins' 2018 https://www.madinamerica.com/2018/01/what-really-call-psychiatric-drugs/
41. http://cepuk.org/unrecognised-facts/no-benefit-over-placebo/
42. https://en.wikipedia.org/wiki/STAR*D
43. http://cepuk.org/unrecognised-facts/no-benefit-over-placebo/
44. https://www.ncbi.nlm.nih.gov/pmc/articles/PMC4172306/

PART 2

45. Arroll B, Chin WY, Moir F, Dowrick C. An evidence-based first consultation for depression: nine key messages. Br J Gen Pract. 2018; 68(669): 200-201. https://doi.org/10.3399/bjgp18X695681 Crossref PubMed Web of Science®Google Scholar
46. Online version: Schuyler, Dean. Depressive spectrum.New York : J. Aronson, [1974] (OCoLC)599454383
47. Posternak MA, 2006, The naturalistic course of unipolar major depression in the absence of somatic therapy, J Nervous and Mental Disease 194: 324-49.
48. http://cepuk.org/unrecognised-facts/long-lasting-negative-effects/
49. https://www.nimh.nih.gov/health/topics/mental-health-medications/index.shtml
50. https://www.counterpunch.org/2014/05/14/psychiatrys-manufacture-of-consent/
51. https://medicatingnormal.com/
52. https://bigthink.com/surprising-science/antidepressant-effects
53. https://popularresistance.org/psychiatrys-manufacture-of-consent-the-antidepressant-explosion/
54. https://patient.info/doctor/screening-for-depression-in-primary-care https://www.bmj.com/content/370/bmj.m3313
55. S. Hyman, "Initiation and adaptation: A paradigm for understanding psychotropic drug action," Am J Psychiatry 153 (1996):151-61.
56. The%20NIMH-funded%20Sequenced%20Treatment%20Alternatives%20to%20Relieve%20Depression,longest%20study%20e ver%20conducted%20to%20evaluate%20depression%20treatment.
57. https://realisticmedicine.scot/the-five-questions/
58. https://psychiatryonline.org/guidelines
59. https://s4be.cochrane.org/start-here/what-is-evidence-based-medicine/

60. https://www.rcpsych.ac.uk/docs/default-source/improving-care/better-mh-policy/position-statements/ps04_19---antidepressants-and-depression.pdf?sfvrsn=ddea9473_5

61. www.cep.org.uk/unrecognised facts

62. https://www.fda.gov/patients/learn-about-expanded-access-and-other-treatment-options/understanding-unapproved-use-approved-drugs-label

63. https://www.medscape.com/viewarticle/864028

64. https://www.bmj.com/content/351/bmj.h5861.full

65. http://cepuk.org/unrecognised-facts/altered-mental-states/

66. https://www.drugawareness.org/tag/candace-pert/

67. https://pubmed.ncbi.nlm.nih.gov/29866014/

68. https://www.eurekaselect.com/162794/article

69. https://medlineplus.gov/druginfo/meds/a699001.html

70. https://medlineplus.gov/antidepressants.html

71. https://www.washingtonpost.com/national/health-science/doctors-often-dont-tell-you-about-drug-side effects-and-thats-a-problem/2017/07/28/830fbaf6-715c-11e7-8839-ec48ec4cae25_story.html

72. https://www.karger.com/Article/FullText/447034

73. https://www.medicines.org.uk/emc/files/pil.6046.pdf

74. https://rxisk.org/experiencing-a-drug-side-effect/

75. https://akathisiaalliance.org/

76. https://davidhealy.org/left-hanging-suicide-in-bridgend/

77. https://rxisk.org/illnesses-worse-than-side effects/

78. https://rxisk.org/akathisia/

79. https://www.missd.co/#:~:text=MISSD%20is%20pleased%20to%20now%20offer%20Akathisia%20101.,Social %20Workers%20for%201%20continuing%20education%20contact%20ho

80. http://breggin.com/studies/Breggin2007.pdf

81. https://www.psycom.net/serotonin-syndrome

82. https://rxisk.org/post-ssri-sexual-dysfunction-pssd/

Bahrick AS. Post SSRI sexual dysfunction. ASAP Tablet. 2006;7(3):2-3,10-11.

Bahrick AS. Persistence of sexual dysfunction side effects after discontinuation of antidepressant medications: Emerging evidence. The Open Psychology Journal. 2008;1:42-50.

83. https://www.health.harvard.edu/womens-health/when-an-ssri-medication-impacts-your-sex-life

84. https://rxisk.org/wp-content/uploads/2015/02/2014-Brookwell-SSRIs-and-Alcohol-JRS616.pdf https://pubmed.ncbi.nlm.nih.gov/23796469/

85. https://rxisk.org/driven-to-drink-antidepressants-and-cravings-for-alcohol/

86. https://rxisk.org/the-dark-is-for-mushrooms-not-for-women/ https://health.usnews.com/health-news/patient-advice/articles/2016-01-13/antidepressants-during-pregnancy-stay-on-them-or-stop

87. https://www.cdc.gov/mmwr/volumes/65/wr/m m6503a1.htm

88. https://womensmentalhealth.org/posts/ssris-and-pphn-the-fda-revises-its-warning/

89. https://jamanetwork.com/journals/jamapediatrics/fullarticle/2476187

90. https://www.cdc.gov/pregnancy/meds/treatingfortwo/features/ssrisandbirthdefects.html

91. http://www.smartcarebhcs.org/important-drug-interactions-with-the-ssris/

92. https://rxisk.org/tools/drug-interaction-checker/

93. https://www.ncbi.nlm.nih.gov/pmc/articles/PMC2771172

94. https://www.sciencedaily.com/releases/2004/12/041203100252.htm

95. https://www.karger.com/Article/Pdf/501215

96. https://akathisiainfo.wordpress.com/2012/03/10/akathisia-info/

97. https://breggin.com/violence-and-suicide-caused-by-antidepressants-report-to-the-fda/

98. https://www.ncbi.nlm.nih.gov/pmc/articles/PMC5061092/

99. http://dx.doi.org/10.15585/mmwr.mm6722a1

100. https://www.weforum.org/agenda/2019/05/the-global-suicide-rate-is-growing-what-can-we-do/

101. https://www.ncbi.nlm.nih.gov/pubmed/19610491

102. www.ssristories.org

103. https://www.nytimes.com/2020/05/19/health/pandemic-coronavirus-suicide-health.html

104. https://www.fda.gov/media/72995/download

105. https://www.nytimes.com/2020/09/07/well/live/prescription-medication-drug-side effects-cascade.html

106. https://www.washingtonpost.com/national/health-science/doctors-often-dont-tell-you-about-drug-side effects-and-thats-a-problem/2017/07/28/830fbaf6-715c-11e7-8839-ec48ec4cae25_story.html

107. https://www.pimsplus.org/about/

108. Serotonin is heavily involved in the 'Fear' (Fight /flight) circuitry https://www.ncbi.nlm.nih.gov/pmc/articles/PMC4820447/

109. https://www.ncbi.nlm.nih.gov/pmc/articles/PMC5864293/

110. https://www.madinamerica.com/2016/11/whats-harm-taking-antidepressant/

111. https://hulpgids.nl/assets/files/pdf/DESS.pdf

112. https://www.psychtools.info/phq15/

113. https://www.apa.org/monitor/2013/07-08/symptoms

114. https://www.bmj.com/content/346/bmj.f1580

115. https://www.bmj.com/content/346/bmj.f1580/rapid-responses

116. cpsych.ac.uk/mental-health/problems-disorders/medically-unexplained-symptoms

117. https://providers.bcidaho.com/resources/pdfs/medical-management/behavioral-health/PHQ-15.pdf

118. https://www.hgi.org.uk/sites/default/files/hgi/Marions%20infographic_for%20print%20A4%20x%202%20page s.pdf

119. https://www.hgi.org.uk/sites/default/files/hgi/Marions%20infographic_for%20print%20A4%20x%202%20page s.pdf

120. https://www.inquirer.com/philly/health/health-news/doctors-dont-provide-enough-information-about-the-side effects-of-drugs-20170802.html

121. https://www.fda.gov/drugs/drug-information-consumers/finding-and-learning-about-side effects-adverse-reactions

122. https://www.accessdata.fda.gov/scripts/medwatch/index.cfm?action=reporting.home

123. https://rxisk.org/about/

124. https://rxisk.org/about/team/

125. https://uk.video.search.yahoo.com/yhs/search;_ylt=AwrIQZydz3VfDZUA2Bl3Bwx.;_ylu=Y29sbwMEcG9zAz EEdnRpZAMEc2VjA3Nj?p=how+to+learn+about+the+adverse+effects+of+medications&fr=yhs-adk-adk_sbnt&hspart=adk&hsimp=yhs-adk_sbnt

126. https://www.madinamerica.com/wp-content/uploads/2017/01/Age-of-Prozac.pdf

127. Posternak MA, 2006, The naturalistic course of unipolar major depression in the absence of somatic therapy, J Nervous and Mental Disease 194: 324-49.

128. https://www.healthline.com/health-news/do-antidepressants-help-in-long-run#Conclusions-are-tough-to-draw

131. http://cepuk.org/unrecognised-facts/long-term-outcomes/

130. https://www.madinamerica.com/author/rwhitaker/

131. Can long-term treatment with antidepressant drugs worsen the course of depression? Fava, G. Journal of Clinical Psychiatry 64 (2003):123-33. https://pdfs.semanticscholar.org/c280/181ab5a63ad93dfdc090eace0d3e0865b6c4.pdf

132. Cartwright C, Gibson K, Read J, Cowan O, Dehar T. Long-term antidepressant use: Patient perspectives of benefits and adverse effects. Patient Prefer Adherence. 2016;10:1401–1407. doi:10.2147/PPA.S110632 https://www.dovepress.com/long-term-antidepressant-use-patient-perspectives-of-benefits-and-adve-peer-reviewed-article-PPA

134. https://news.sky.com

135. https://news.sky.com/story/long-term-use-of-antidepressants-could-cause-permanent-damage-doctors-warn-11688430

135. https://journals.sagepub.com/doi/full/10.1177/2045125320921694

136. http://breggin.com/wp-content/uploads/2012/01/Breggin2011_ChronicBrainImpairment.pdf International Journal of Risk & Safety in Medicine, 23: 193-200)

137. https://www.ncbi.nlm.nih.gov/pmc/articles/PMC5347943/?fbclid=IwAR1B6cNzkvCPBRwQyI8VxbDSxHIq45 R82jqeTLgNjhRDrrr3-qPR-VUXTG8 https://pubmed.ncbi.nlm.nih.gov/28029715/

138. https://www.bmj.com/content/361/bmj.k1315

139. https://uk.finance.yahoo.com/news/antidepressants-taken-millions-significantly-increase-dementia-risk-

140. https://pubmed.ncbi.nlm.nih.gov/24502860/

141. https://care.diabetesjournals.org/content/early/2020/02/12/dc19-1175

142. https://www.madnessradio.net/files/tardivedysphoriadarticle.pdf

143. https://www.psychologytoday.com/us/blog/mad-in-america/201106/now-antidepressant-induced-chronic-depression-has-name-tardive-dysphoria

144. https://www.midcitiespsychiatry.com/treatment-resistant-depression/

145. https://pubmed.ncbi.nlm.nih.gov/22654508/

146. https://en.wikipedia.org/wiki/Antidepressant_treatment_tachyphylaxis

147. https://www.healthyplace.com/depression/antidepressants/do-antidepressants-lose-their-effect

148. https://www.letstalkwithdrawal.com/category/blog/

149. https://www.drugabuse.gov/publications/media-guide/science-drug-use-addiction-basics#

150. https://www.nytimes.com/2018/04/07/health/antidepressants-withdrawal-prozac-cymbalta.html

151. https://www.bma.org.uk/what-we-do/population-health/prescription-and-illicit-drugs/prescribed-drugs-associated-with-dependence-and-withdrawal

152. https://www.health.harvard.edu/blog/millions-skip-medications-due-to-their-high-cost-201501307673

153. https://www.thenation.com/article/society/mental-health-insurance-coronavirus/

154. https://www.ctvnews.ca/health/canadians-warn-of-self-harm-risk-amid-severe-shortage-of-antidepressant-drug-1.5200797

155. http://www.parliament.scot/S5_PublicPetitionsCommittee/Submissions%20 2018/PE1651_TTTTTTT.pdf

156. https://www.psychiatrictimes.com/view/impoverishment-psychiatric-knowledge

157. https://pubmed.ncbi.nlm.nih.gov/32435449/

158. http://www.antidepressantsfacts.com/effexor-withdrawal6.htm

159. https://www.nytimes.com/2011/07/10/opinion/sunday/10antidepressants.html?pagewanted=all

160. https://www.psychologytoday.com/us/blog/sideeffects/201107/antidepressant-withdrawal-syndrome

161. Batelaan NM, Bosman RC, Muntingh A, Scholten WD, Huijbregts KM, van Balkom AJLM.

    Risk of relapse after antidepressant discontinuation in anxiety disorders, obsessive-compulsive disorder, and post-traumatic stress disorder: systematic review and meta-analysis of relapse prevention trials. BMJ. 2017;358:j3927.

162. The British Journal of Psychiatry (2020) Page 1 of 4. doi: 10.1192/bjp.2019.269

    https://pharmaceutical-journal.com/article/news/nice-amends-depression-guideline-highlighting-severe-and-long-lasting-withdrawal-symptoms

    https://www.pulsetoday.co.uk/news/clinical-areas/prescribing/nice-antidepressant-withdrawal-guidance-misleading-and-without-evidence/

163. https://pubmed.ncbi.nlm.nih.gov/30292574/

164. https://www.cambridge.org/core/journals/epidemiology-and-psychiatric-sciences/article/antidepressant-withdrawal-the-tide-is-finally-turning/8394C10FE317CA5A39B62B86793FC3ED

165. https://www.psychologytoday.com/us/blog/sideeffects/201908/antidepressant-withdrawal-and-scientific-consensus

166. https://www.ncbi.nim.nih.gov/pmc/articles/PMC8061160/

167. https://www.cambridge.org/core/journals/epidemiology-and-psychiatric-sciences/article/antidepressant-withdrawal-the-tide-is-finally-turning/8394C10FE317CA5A39B62B86793FC3ED/core-reader https://www.madinamerica.com/2020/01/researchers-antidepressant-withdrawal-not-discontinuation-syndrome/

168. https://en.wikipedia.org/wiki/Wicked_problem

169. https://withdrawal.theinnercompass.org/learn/primer-psychiatric-drug-dependence-tolerance-and-withdrawal

170. https://www.psychiatrictimes.com/view/international-antidepressant-withdrawal-crisis-time-act

171. https://www.thelancet.com/journals/lanpsy/article/PIIS2215-0366(19)30032-X/fulltext

172. https://www.pharmaceutical-journal.com/news-and-analysis/opinion/insight/antidepressant-withdrawal-can-be-a-horrible-experience-are-tapering-strips-a-potential-solution/20207867.fullarticle?firstPass=false

173. https://www.thelancet.com/journals/lanpsy/article/PIIS2215-0366(19)30032-X/fulltext

174. https://bpspubs.onlinelibrary.wiley.com/doi/full/10.1111/bcp.14475

175. https://bpspubs.onlinelibrary.wiley.com/doi/10.1111/

176. https://www.southampton.ac.uk/medicine/academic_units/projects/reduce.page#project_overview%0A

177. https://medicine.unimelb.edu.au/research-groups/general-practice-research/mental-health-program/wiserad-a-randomised-trial-of-a-structured-online-intervention-to-promote-and-support-antidepressant-de-prescribing-in-primary-care

178. https://www.umcg.nl/EN/corporate/News/Paginas/first-patient-discontinuation-antidepressants.aspx

179. https://www.thelancet.com/journals/lanpsy/article/PIIS2215-0366(19)30032-X/fulltext

180. https://www.taperingstrip.com/

181. https://journals.sagepub.com/doi/10.1177/2045125320954609

182. https://www.taperingstrip.com/prescribing-and-ordering/?q=

PART 3

183. Hall, W. (2012). Harm reduction guide to coming off psychiatric drugs and withdrawal (2nd ed.). The Icarus Project and Freedom Centre

184. http://willhall.net/comingoffmeds/

185. https://www.theinnercompass.org/learn-unlearn/intervention/antidepressants

186. https://withdrawal.theinnercompass.org/taper

https://withdrawal.theinnercompass.org/taper/twps-key-withdrawal-related-information-fda-approved-drug-label

187. https://www.madinamerica.com/2013/08/ssri-discontinuation-is-even-more-problematic-than-acknowledged/

188. https://rxisk.org/protracted-antidepressant-withdrawal/

189. https://withdrawal.theinnercompass.org/page/withdrawal-symptoms-z

190. https://prescribeddrug.info/

191. https://www.nytimes.com/2019/03/05/health/depression-withdrawal-drugs.html https://www.psychologytoday.com/us/blog/side effects/201810/antidepressant-withdrawal-said-affect-millions

https://iipdw.org/royal-college-of-psychiatrists-changes-its-position-on-antidepressant-withdrawal/

192. https://psychiatryonline.org/pb/assets/raw/sitewide/practice_guidelines/guidelines/mdd.pdf

193. https://www.rcpsych.ac.uk/mental-health/treatments-and-wellbeing/stopping-antidepressants https://www.pharmaceutical-journal.com/news-and-analysis/news/national-guidance-for-antidepressant-withdrawal-too-fast-for-some-patients-says-rcpsych/20206614.article?firstPass=false

https://www.rcpsych.ac.uk/news-and-features/latest-news/detail/2020/09/23/new-information-on-stopping-antidepressants

194. https://www.bma.org.uk/what-we-do/population-health/prescription-and-illicit-drugs/prescribed-drugs-associated-with-dependence-and-withdrawal

195. https://www.michaelwest.com.au/websites-research-online-advice-on-medications-skewed-by-big-pharma-funding/

196. https://content.iospress.com/articles/international-journal-of-risk-and-safety-in-medicine/jrs191023

197. https://americanaddictioncenters.org/withdrawal-timelines-treatments/anti-depressants

198. https://www.madinamerica.com/2013/08/ssri-discontinuation-is-even-more-problematic-than-acknowledged/

PART 4

199. https://www.statista.com/statistics/205042/proportion-of-brand-to-generic-prescriptions-dispensed/

200. (Rosenthal, Jessica & Kong, Brian & Jacobs, Leslie & Katzman, Martin. (2008) The Journal of family practice. 57. 109-14.)

201. https://www.newstatesman.com/spotlight/healthcare/2020/05/why-mental-health-human-right

202. Selective serotonin reuptake inhibitors in childhood depression. Whittington, C. The Lancet 363 (2004):1341-5.

203. https://www.fda.gov/drugs/postmarket-drug-safety-information-patients-and-providers/suicidality-children-and-adolescents-being-treated-antidepressant-medications

204. https://www.fda.gov/consumers/consumer-updates/fda-dont-leave-childhood-depression-untreated

205. https://www.verywellmind.com/should-children-take-antidepressants-

206. http://info.1in5minds.org/blog/7-free-screening-tools-for-childrens-mental-health-concerns#:~

207. https://www.madinamerica.com/antidepressants-pediatric-use/

208. ews.curtin.edu.au/media-releases/research-reveals-alarming-link-between-rising-antidepressant-use-and-suicide-rates-among-young-australians/?utm_source=miragenews&utm_medium=miragenews&utm_campaign=news

209. https://www.wix.app/blog/post/5f98d1f2b616490017b79f82?metaSiteId=e46126be-5e83-4973-a0fe-598613447990&d=https://www.psychwatchaustralia.com/post/melbourne-s-covid-spike-in-antidepressant-use-may-trigger-suicides-by-children-and-adolescents?postId%3D5f98d1f2b616490017b79f82

210. A. Martin. "Age effects on antidepressant-induced manic conversion," Arch of Pediatrics & Adolescent Medicine(2002) 158: 773-80.

211. https://www.fda.gov/drugs/postmarket-drug-safety-information-patients-and-providers/suicidality-children-and-adolescents-being-treated-antidepressant-medications

212. Bartels, Stephen et al. Evidence-Based Practices in Geriatric Mental Health in Psychiatric Services, November 2002. http://www.ps.psychiatryonline.org/cgi/content/full/53/11/1419

213. Arthur, A., Savva, G. M., Barnes, L. E., Borjian-Boroojeny, A., Dening, T., Jagger, C., . . . & the Cognitive Function and Ageing Studies Collaboration. (2019). Changing prevalence and treatment of depression among older people over two decades. The British Journal of Psychiatry. doi: 10.1192/bjp.2019.193

214. https://www.bmj.com/content/343/bmj.d4551 Coupland, Carol et al. "Antidepressant use and risk of adverse outcomes in older people: population based cohort study" in BMJ, August 2, 2011. http://www.bmj.com/content/343/bmj.d4551

215. Arthur, A., Savva, G. M., Barnes, L. E., Borjian-Boroojeny, A., Dening, T., Jagger, C., . . . & the Cognitive Function and Ageing Studies Collaboration. (2019). Changing prevalence and treatment of depression among older people over two decades. The British Journal of Psychiatry. doi: 10.1192/bjp.2019.193

216. Weigand AJ, Bondi MW, Thomas KR, Campbell NL, Galasko DR, Salmon DP, . . . & Delano-Wood L. (2020). Association of anticholinergic medication and AD biomarkers with incidence of MCI among cognitively normal older adults. Neurology. Published online September 2, 2020. DOI: 10.1212/WNL.0000000000010643

217. DLinx (January 2019). https://www.mdlinx.com/internal-medicine/article/3272.

218. https://www.psychologytoday.com/us/blog/envy/201902/loneliness-new-epidemic-in-the-usa#:~:text=Loneliness%20affects%20almost%20half%20of%20adult%20Americans.%20Loneliness,adults%E 2%80%94double%20the%20number%20affected%20a%20few%20decades%20ago.

219. https://www.nia.nih.gov/health/depression-and-older-adults

220. https://www.brainline.org/article/ptsd-fact-sheet-frequently-asked-questions

221. Forbes D, Creamer M, Phelps A, et al. Australian Guidelines for the Treatment of Adults with Acute Stress Disorder and Post-traumatic Stress Disorder. Aust N Z J Psychiatry. 2007;41:637–648. [PubMed] [Google Scholar]

222. https://www.ptsd.va.gov/professional/treat/cooccurring/index.asp

223. https://www.ncbi.nlm.nih.gov/pmc/articles/PMC5047000/

224. https://www.ptsd.va.gov/professional/assessment/screens/pc-ptsd.asp

225. https://www.madinamerica.com/2019/11/screening-drug-treatment-increase-veteran-suicides/

226. https://www.washingtonpost.com/opinions/2020/09/17/im-veteran-who-was-suicidal-its-good-thing-i-didnt-have-access-gun/

227. https://www.huffingtonpost.co.uk/entry/veterans-ptsd-marijuana_n_7506760?ri18n=true

228. https://www.madinamerica.com/veterans-2/

229. https://www.warfighteradvance.org/

230. https://afsp.org/

PART 5

231. https://www.psychologytoday.com/us/blog/the-inertia-trap/201304/how-pharmaceutical-ads-distort-healthcare-markets

232. https://www.nytimes.com/2017/12/24/business/media/prescription-drugs-advertising-tv.html

233. https://www.biopharmadive.com/news/pharma-ad-dtc-marketing-2018-spend-TV-congress/533319

234. https://cdn1.sph.harvard.edu/wp-content/uploads/sites/94/2016/05/STAT-Harvard-Poll-May-2016-FDA-Regulation.pdf

235. https://www.psychologytoday.com/us/blog/side effects/201605/the-effort-rid-tv-pharma-ads

236. https://www.scientificamerican.com/article/this-drug-ad-is-not-right-for-you/

237. http://www.parliament.scot/GettingInvolved/Petitions/PE01651

238. https://journals.sagepub.com/doi/pdf/10.1177/2045125320967183

239. https://www.madinamerica.com/2020/12/listening-patient-voice-antidepressant-withdrawal-experience/

240. https://reliefweb.int/sites/reliefweb.int/files/resources/G1707604.p

241. https://mhanational.org/b4stage4-philosophy

242. https://www.nytimes.com/2009/10/22/health/22nami.html

243. Batt, S., Butler, J., Shannon, O. et al. Pharmaceutical Ethics and Grassroots Activism in the United States: A Social History Perspective. Bioethical Inquiry 17, 49–60 (2020). https://doi.org/10.1007/s11673-019-09956-8

244. https://www.360marketupdates.com/global-antidepressants-market-12883580

245. https://www.theguardian.com/world/2020/mar/25/why-its-healthy-to-be-afraid-in-a-crisis

246. https://www.collaborativemedconsulting.com/single-post/2020/04/10/Mental-illness-is-not-a-disease-and-therefore-cannot-be-an-epidemic-but-unless-we-challenge-the-current-mental-health-narrative-%E2%80%98Memories-of-times-past-will-speak-to-the-present-and-project-on-to-the-unknown-future

247. https://undocs.org/A/HRC/44/48

248. https://www.bma.org.uk/what-we-do/population-health/prescription-and-illicit-drugs/prescribed-drugs-associated-with-dependence-and-withdrawal

249. https://www.fda.gov/drugs/information-consumers-and-patients-drugs/finding-and-learning-about-side-effects-adverse-reactions